☀ THE BEGINNER'S GUIDE TO ☽
EGO DEATH

THE BEGINNER'S GUIDE TO
EGO DEATH

AJ MURILLO

EXPAND YOUR MIND THROUGH PSYCHEDELIC EXPLORATION

ULYSSES PRESS

Published by:
Ulysses Press
PO Box 3440
Berkeley, CA 94703
www.ulyssespress.com

ISBN: 978-1-64604-789-5
Library of Congress Control Number: 2024944974

Printed in the United States
10 9 8 7 6 5 4 3 2 1

Acquisitions editor: Shelona Belfon
Managing editor: Claire Chun
Project editor: Renee Rutledge
Proofreader: Beret Olsen
Front cover design: David Hastings
Interior artwork: pages 20, 109, 173, 187, and 203 ©Kateryna Maltseva; remaining graphics from shutterstock.com: page 15 © agsandrew, page 68 © AntonKhrupinArt, page 75 © imagewriter, page 78 © Adam Chai, page 84 © ilusmedical, page 121 © Bruce Rolff, page 147 © Titima Ongkantong, page 153 © Jorm Sangsorn, page 179 © PsychedelicArt
Interior design: Winnie Liu
Layout: Jake Flaherty Design

IMPORTANT NOTE TO READERS: This book has been written and published for informational and educational purposes only. It is not intended to serve as medical advice or to be any form of medical treatment. You should always consult with your physician before altering or changing any aspect of your medical treatment. Do not stop or change any prescription medications without the guidance and advice of your physician. Any use of the information in this book is made on the reader's good judgment and is the reader's sole responsibility. This book is not intended to diagnose or treat any medical condition and is not a substitute for a physician. This book is independently authored and published and no sponsorship or endorsement of this book by, and no affiliation with, any trademarked brands or other products mentioned within is claimed or suggested. All trademarks that appear in this book belong to their respective owners and are used here for informational purposes only. The author and publisher encourage readers to patronize the brands mentioned in this book.

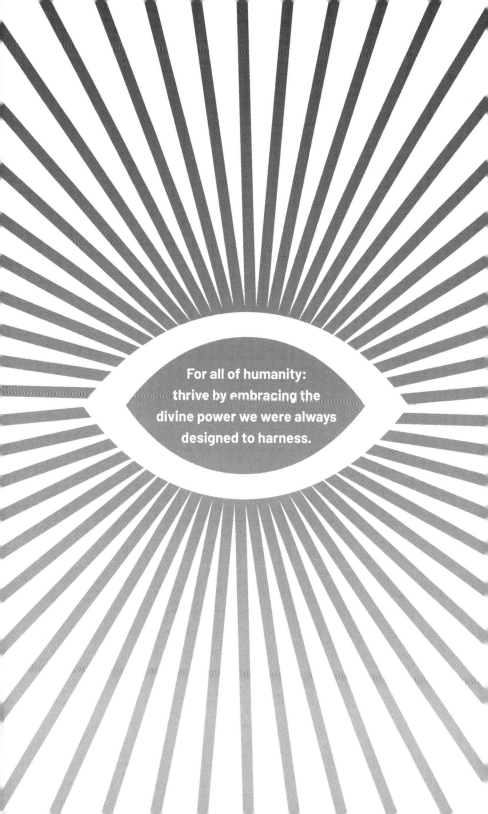

For all of humanity:
thrive by embracing the
divine power we were always
designed to harness.

CONTENTS

PREFACE	ix
WHO AM I?	1
INTRODUCTION: STEPPING OUT OF THE "NORM" & INTO THE UNKNOWN	3
PART 1: HUMAN EXPERIENCE 101	**15**
CHAPTER 1: THE PSYCHE	16
CHAPTER 2: PERSONALITY PERCEPTION	43
CHAPTER 3: REALITY	64
CHAPTER 4: THE JOURNEY OF THE SOUL	110
PART 2: EGO DEATH—CHARTING THE COURSE TO SELF-REBIRTH	**121**
CHAPTER 5: ALIGNING PSYCHEDELIC CHOICES WITH GOALS	122
CHAPTER 6: PREPARING FOR THE JOURNEY	141
CHAPTER 7: LEVEL 1 EGO DEATH	157
CHAPTER 8: LEVEL 3 EGO DEATH: THE THIRD-EYE AWAKENING	174
CHAPTER 9: LEVEL 2 EGO DEATH	188
CHAPTER 10: LIFE AFTER DEATH	204
CHAPTER 11: FINAL WORDS	213
BIBLIOGRAPHY	216
INDEX	217
ACKNOWLEDGMENTS	225
ABOUT THE AUTHOR	227

PREFACE

The mysteries of life remain, even as millennia of human evolution unfold. Our journey has been marked by remarkable achievements—yet, amidst our progress, profound questions about existence persist. What does it mean to truly live? Why do we exist? How do we attain genuine happiness and liberation in a world fraught with complexities?

Since ancient times, we've harnessed chemical power to shape our reality—prioritizing it over the potential of the mind itself. From the earliest weaponization, humanity has shown a relentless focus on mastering the external world, driven by survival instincts and a quest for dominance. Science and technology, our modern tools of advancement, have propelled us forward, yet our inner evolution—our understanding of purpose and fulfillment—lags behind. It is as though we have become adept at navigating the external world while neglecting the depths of our own consciousness—the one thing we truly all have in common.

In our pursuit of survival and material wealth, the true essence of our existence often remains obscured. We find ourselves amidst a paradox: in an age of unprecedented knowledge and innovation, a persistent struggle to harness the full potential of our minds continues.

Without diving into the profound curiosities and fundamental questions about our existence, life remains in a state of imbalance. And a world where individuals are imbalanced—oblivious to their purpose and potential—is destined for chaos.

In a perfect world, every human would embrace their soul's journey. They'd recognize their life's purpose through a profound connection with the universe, forging an unbreakable bond that stretches beyond the limits of the material world. By embracing this sacred connection, they would unlock the true potential of their minds as they become aware of the seamless connection between infinite intelligence and themselves. This divine relationship would illuminate their path, guiding them to embrace the present moment with unwavering clarity. In this state of heightened awareness, they would come to realize the untapped reservoir of creativity, insight, and intuition waiting to be unleashed. Like a master sculptor shaping clay, they would mold the raw material of their thoughts and emotions into vessels of creation. With hearts as open as the skies, they would dance with the winds of change, navigating the sway and motions of life, effortlessly. With their true power ignited and their unique talents embraced, they'd glide through life's complexities with grace—transcending obstacles that dared to obstruct their path—ultimately fulfilling their destiny. And in the embrace of emotional intelligence and empathy, they would bridge the chasm between souls, transcending the superficial boundaries that divide humanity.

I know; sounds pretty far-fetched, doesn't it? I mean, I did mention "in a perfect world." The truth is far from utopia. Instead, we find so many people still feeling disconnected from their souls. Our true reality remains full of chaos, confusion, and widespread suffering. In the heart of destruction, negativity has taken root, shaping the world as we know it. Brokenness and pain seem to saturate every corner of existence, dimming the beauty of life.

Ironically, these aspects of life are inevitable—they are the yin to life's yang, the shadow to its light. What makes this situation insufferable is not the existence of these challenges but the overwhelming dominance they hold over our world. Realistically, destruction is often a necessary precursor to creation, a fundamental aspect of the natural order. The concept of yin and yang beautifully illustrates this truth. It is through negativity that we learn to recognize and cultivate positivity, finding strength in adversity and wisdom in struggle. Life's elaborate design demands a delicate balance between creation and destruction, a balance that can only be achieved through a profound knowledge of self. Our downfall as a collective lies in our lack of this self-awareness. We fall short of understanding the bigger picture of life, and this ignorance is exploited by those who run the world, leading us into the same destructive patterns generation after generation. At the root of this ignorance is the ego—an invisible force that shapes our lives without our awareness. It thrives in the absence of self-knowledge, subtly trapping us and steering both our individual and collective realities. Only through ego death and a deep understanding of the self can we hope to manifest positive change.

WHO AM I?

I am AJ "the Sage" Murillo and honored to be your guide. As a seemingly ordinary human, I've been entrusted with a divine life purpose: to articulate the complexities of our multidimensional human existence. My goal is to provide a clear and accessible understanding of our human design and help you navigate your unique life path by harnessing the full power we were all meant to access.

Throughout my life, I've received strange and divine signs—glimpses into the future and reality-bending experiences—that made me realize there's far more to our existence than just the physical world we see. These experiences were like puzzle pieces, guiding me toward the understanding of my true purpose. But it wasn't until I experienced psychedelic journeys and ego death breakthroughs that I was able to fully understand and integrate all of this. These experiences allowed me to reconnect with my soul on a deep level, revealing ancient knowledge I've carried with me for lifetimes. This journey has been intense, but it's allowed me to understand the full spectrum of our human experience and design. I've gained a deep understanding of how the human psyche operates—not just my own mind, but the intricacies of our collective existence.

Through my personal journey, I've managed to navigate through the elaborate labyrinth of consciousness, staying present and introspective during my psychedelic voyages. These experiences allowed me to unravel the fabric of our existence and gain a deeper understanding of what consciousness truly entails. From understanding life at its highest peaks to its deepest depths, I've anchored this knowledge in a way that's not just understandable but actionable.

Now, it's my privilege to share these insights with you, guiding you toward your own ego death—an experience that will allow you to access deeper parts of yourself and gain the clarity needed to navigate your unique journey with confidence and purpose.

STEPPING OUT OF THE "NORM" & INTO THE UNKNOWN

Welcome to *The Beginner's Guide to Ego Death*—a paradoxical journey into the depths of self-discovery and liberation Whether you're embarking on your first steps toward an ego death journey or preparing to deepen your awakening, this marks a pivotal moment—a crossroads where you answer the call of your soul.

It's funny, isn't it? The thought of an ego death is something most people instinctively would shy away from. The word "ego" is often met with discomfort and misconceptions. Some people believe it's irrelevant, dismissing it as something reserved for self-centered maniacs. Others vaguely avoid this subject, uncomfortable with acknowledging parts of themselves they prefer to keep hidden. Many individuals don't know themselves well enough to even consider the complexities of their psyche, let alone wake up thinking about their ego or desiring its demise. Yet, despite its initial strangeness, ego deaths hold a profound potential for positive and life-altering transformation. While it may evoke fear or uncertainty at first glance, digging deeper reveals the hidden gems of wisdom within.

On one hand, ego death is this deep dive into the depths of your own mind, where you're confronting fears head-on and coming face-to-face with uncomfortable truths. It's a process of peeling back layers of yourself, shedding parts of who you thought you were to uncover the essence of your true self. But here lies the heart of the matter: in the midst of this journey toward the "death" of certain parts of ourselves, we're actually opening ourselves up to life in its fullest. We release what no longer serves us and make room for new growth, new possibilities, and a deeper connection with the world around us, as well as the entirety of our existence.

But, let's be honest, for many—the idea of facing something heavy and deep can be more intimidating than exciting—right?

I mean, think about it, many of us tend to avoid anything that might unsettle us emotionally. We're often so caught up in our day-to-day routines, sticking to what's comfortable and familiar. So when it comes to exploring the unknown—whether it's in our minds or out there in the world—it can feel incredibly uncomfortable navigating through uncharted territory.

It's like venturing into the wilderness without a map, not knowing what you'll find or where you'll end up. It's safe to say that it can be a significant anxiety trigger. In our everyday lives, it's normal for the uncharted depths of our minds and the unexplored reaches of our realities to remain untouched. So, in contrast, the journey of an ego death represents a brave departure from the norm—a deliberate exploration into the depths of the wilderness of our own consciousness.

It's a thought-provoking realization that our own minds can feel like unfamiliar territory, and even more so that it has become our norm to remain outsiders within ourselves. This perspective really makes you think about the concept of normalcy and ponder the idea that what we label as "the norm"—the familiar set of beliefs and behaviors shaped by your personal experiences and upbringing—isn't necessarily good or bad; it's more like a familiar routine, something we're used to without even realizing it. It's so ingrained that we hardly even question or examine it.

Of course, having some structure in our lives can be comforting and necessary. It brings a sense of order and familiarity. However, there's a subtle yet significant difference between the normalcy of our daily routines and the normalcy of leaving aspects of our minds and lives unexplored.

It's this very structure that becomes a barrier in the flow of life. This barrier can keep us from venturing into new realms of possibility and experiencing life's wonders, preventing our souls from evolving and keeping us from fully embracing the magic that life has to offer.

WHAT I LEARNED FROM MY FIRSTHAND EGO DEATH EXPERIENCE

During an ego death experience on an LSD journey, I uncovered a profound truth about our realities. It wasn't just about how our minds construct these realities through our personality, emotions, and experiences. I also realized that our realities are default settings handed to us by our circumstances. We find ourselves committed to playing a specific character or role within this pre-defined reality.

This was an unforgettable trip. I settled into a comfortable position. Engulfed in the ethereal tones of supernatural frequencies, I surrendered to the rhythm, letting my mind merge with the music. And then, in a sudden flash of insight, it all became clear. It was as if I could physically see that there was infinite space beyond my immediate reality. During that profound moment, time seemed to slow to a standstill, and the scene before me became more than just what my eyes could perceive. I saw my life laid out like a scene from a movie, every detail vivid and clear—who I was, what I was doing, where I lived, every choice I had made, encapsulating my entire being in a single moment. It felt as if I were merely a spectator, watching myself from a distance, while beyond this singular scene lay an expanse of infinite space. My little reality appeared as a mere speck in the vastness of the universe.

As I zoomed into the details of my reality, a character emerged— one who had settled into a life that didn't quite align with their true happiness, yet continued to play this role nonetheless, navigating the ups and downs as they came. It was a scene depicting choices lived out, choices that felt uncomfortably normal, showcasing struggles and moments of defeat. This experience allowed me to recognize the clear patterns in my thinking that were keeping me tethered to a specific reality. However, it was in witnessing this scene that the realization dawned—had I not seen this, I wouldn't have recognized the depth of my choices or the patterns I had fallen into. I would have continued living, understanding my life only as I saw it, unaware of the underlying narratives shaping my existence. In that moment of observation, the spectator within me couldn't help but wonder: How can they even fathom living beyond this reality when they can't see or understand that there is a life outside of it? This is their world, their perspective—what they know and what they see. This marked the beginning of my realization that I had been living on a default setting, unaware and somewhat lost within its confines.

As I explored beyond my personal reality, I marveled at the vastness of space that surrounded my tiny slice of existence. It dawned on me that just as there are dimensions within ourselves—ways we think and perceive—similarly, the external reality is equally vast and multidimensional. Each of us occupies a realm entirely our own, a tiny speck amidst the vast expanse of infinite space. Yet, within this humble space, lies a universe of opportunities waiting to be embraced, opportunities to expand our realities outward.

As I swallowed this information, it felt like trying to hold the entire universe in my hands—it was almost overwhelming. While this perspective seemed crystal clear to the observer within me, I discovered that my lower self, the character I embody, initially had difficulty fully digesting and making sense of it all. Yet, as I absorbed and processed this knowledge, I found it to be a profound game changer. It was as simple as realizing that life is like a stage, and we're all playing various roles. Every moment, every scene, offers us the chance to savor life on our own terms. But, without this awareness, we wouldn't truly live on our terms but according to what we perceive as our reality, influenced by our circumstances, hence, leading to what can be termed as the default reality.

However, I soon realized that while this insight may sound straightforward, its depth goes beyond words, and many may struggle to fully comprehend it without experiencing it themselves. This is why I often make it a point to find tangible and relatable ways to tether this profound wisdom gained from my psychedelic journeys with everyday experiences, making it accessible for everyone to understand the unseen magic of our human existence.

Switching the Channel of Your Reality

So, imagine your mind as a box, like a television or a screen projector. This box plays a channel of reality—your reality—but here's the twist: you don't realize you're watching a channel, let alone that you're the projector itself, because you're too busy being the main character. You find yourself tuned into the same show repeatedly, familiar with its plots and characters because it's what your psyche and personality gravitate toward. These internal dynamics play out certain narratives, sometimes intriguing and captivating, while other times mundane or even unsettling, depending on the lens through which you view them. It's like being an actor in your own life story, playing out scenes that can be humorous, sorrowful, suspenseful, or heartwarming, all influenced by the complex relationship between your character's psyche, background story, and personality traits. This is the channel that has been gifted to you, your default reality. Now, imagine the hidden gem you're seeking: it's like finding the remote control to your entire reality. With it, you're not just passively going along with what life or society has taught you—you have the power to change the channel. You could switch between different experiences, perspectives, and realities, shaping your life with intention rather than letting external circumstances dictate it.

RECLAIMING YOUR POWER

Simply wanting to change your life by thinking about it isn't enough. The psyche is far more complex than it appears. We're made up of layers—different parts of ourselves that have formed throughout our journey, shaping our reality in intricate ways. You can't just change one part of your life and expect everything else to fall into place. There are many sides to who we are, some that need more attention and others we might not even be aware of. These hidden parts often shape what we prioritize or neglect in our reality, steering the direction of our lives without us fully realizing it. That's why an ego death is so important. Ego death isn't just a mental shift—it's like pressing reset on your entire being, allowing you to confront all those layers and the patterns that have unconsciously driven your life path.

Navigating these layers through an ego death allows you to deeply transform how you understand yourself and your reality. Once you experience this, you unlock the ability to truly harness the power within and begin living life on your own terms.

What do I mean by living life on your own terms? Consider how much of your reality is shaped by your mindset. How often are your actions and decisions influenced by thoughts lingering from your mind or emotions rooted in your heart?

These patterns have become second nature, almost automatic. Are they truly yours, or shaped by beliefs and influences you've absorbed unconsciously? How much of your life is guided by these unseen forces, limiting your full potential and exploration of who you truly are?

By daring to challenge and break free from these limiting beliefs and think outside our "norm box," we unlock new dimensions of ourselves—dimensions brimming with untapped creativity, resilience, and possibility.

This is where the words "ego" and "death" take on a whole new meaning. They're not just ideas to fear or shy away from—they are gateways to profound insights and transformative experiences that lie beyond the confines of the norm.

Understanding the power of the ego is to grasp the essence of self-control (control of the self and its reality), while understanding death is to appreciate the preciousness of life itself. So, don't be deterred by the stigma surrounding these words; rather, see them as gateways towards your higher self.

BEYOND HEALING

While there are plenty of great, data-driven psychedelic books showcasing the potential and safety of psychedelic experiences for healing trauma—offered by esteemed PhDs and MDs sharing respected and proven research in their endeavor to aid humanity—this book takes the subject a step further.

It's true, psychedelics can really help us face and heal those deep-rooted traumas that seem to have a grip on how we think, act, and live. But here's the thing—the journey of transformation doesn't stop at healing. Our traumas love to stick around, dictating our every move. While psychedelics prove to be ideal tools for heightened awareness, the journey of transformation extends far beyond mere recognition and healing. Healing may mend the heart, but what about the mind, and that tender relationship that they share?

Yes, our minds may be immensely powerful, but they are also equally delicate. The scars from our past can hide beneath the surface, quietly steering our perceptions of the world and ourselves. Many people think emotional healing is simply about acknowledging pain and moving beyond it, but true healing runs much deeper. That's where psychedelics come in. Psychedelics are truly a gift that grants us a unique opportunity to explore the mental, emotional, and spiritual layers of ourselves, revealing how each aspect influences our lives. With this knowledge, you can do more than heal—you can learn how to step out of your past's shadow and take full control of your life in a more empowered way. Through heightened clarity and awareness, psychedelics allow you to glimpse the intangible and metaphysical aspects of life that shape your existence. Gaining this deeper awareness empowers you to see all corners of your life much more clearly, creating space for personal transformation and true growth. However, you'll need to confidently comprehend what you're experiencing to unlock the full potential of your psychedelic journey. The psychedelic trip offers a glimpse into the higher dimensional aspects of life, revealing realms of consciousness and insights that are vastly different from our everyday experiences. Psychedelics can show you the way, but the real work lies entirely in your hands. While it may feel liberating and eye-opening during the trip, you'll still need to work through the maze of your mind to make those changes truly stick in your life.

THE FOCUS OF THIS GUIDE

In this guide, you'll dive into the complexities of the human psyche and the fundamental truths that govern our reality. You'll explore every angle of yourself, including how your energy shapes your reality. You'll learn to recognize the subtle ways your ego operates, what it takes to dismantle its influence, and how to harness the power within you to break free from its control. I'll lead you towards the threshold of ego death, but I won't leave you stranded there. Instead, I'll provide you with the tools and insights to navigate life after this enlightening experience. This book serves as a bridge—a bridge that connects your highest self, experienced through psychedelics, with your everyday self that intends to grow, heal, and evolve.

This ego death journey is the start of allowing yourself to live freely and authentically as the creator of your own reality. But first, to really experience an ego death, you've got to dig deep into every part of yourself—your character, your life, your mind—and how you see the world. This exploration will teach you how to harness your experiences and emotions as powerful catalysts for profound and lasting change. This journey isn't just about moving forward or coping; it's about taking back control and growing stronger with newfound wisdom as your armor.

Now, as we step onto this path together, we'll embark on the first leg of our journey. In Part 1 of this book, you will gain insights that will reshape your understanding of self and existence. As we continue this journey, Part 2 of the book will serve as a detailed guide to navigating your psychedelic experiences. I will recommend specific psychedelics for accessing different aspects of your psyche, achieving various levels of ego death, and mastering your experiences.

PART I

HUMAN EXPERIENCE 101

The Psyche, Personality Perception, Reality & the Journey of the Soul

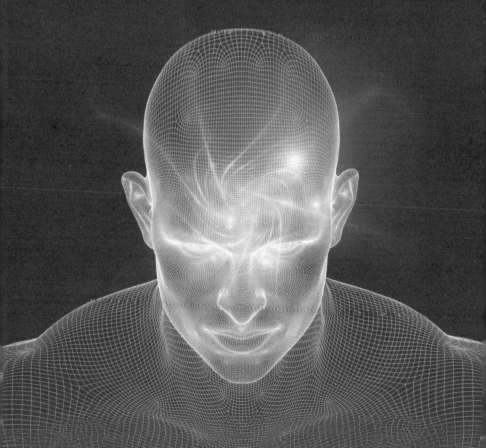

CHAPTER 1

✳ ☽ ✳

THE PSYCHE

To understand the fundamental operations of your mind, you need to understand your thought processes. A significant part of your ego death journey will involve learning to flow with your thoughts. Now, that might sound straightforward, but it actually requires a great deal of focus and self-awareness. The psyche, intertwined and partnered with the emotional guidance system, forms a complex labyrinth that can feel impossible to navigate. Let me emphasize that it may feel impossible at times, but rest assured, it isn't. The key lies in grasping the ego's role in your life and understanding how it shapes your thinking.

WHAT AND WHO IS THE EGO ANYWAY?

It's natural to focus on certain aspects of your identity while overlooking others. We tend to focus on the aspects that are convenient or comfortable, but how truthful and transparent are you about who you really are? How deeply can you honestly examine yourself? How much weight do you place on your self-image?

The invisible force of self-perception, delicately nestled between your thoughts and emotions, offers just a glimpse into understanding your ego's presence.

Before we dive deeper, let's lay the groundwork by discussing the inner workings of your psyche.

Talking about the psyche without mentioning Professor Sigmund Freud seems nearly impossible. It's like trying to discuss modern physics without mentioning Einstein. Interestingly, I stumbled upon my own findings before diving into Freud's theories. It's been quite a journey. I didn't just read about the mind; through psychedelic trips on psilocybin mushrooms and LSD, I experienced firsthand this incredible exploration of our existence. It was like peering behind the curtains of reality, gaining insight into the profound design of our nature and the flow of our existence.

These experiences allowed me to grasp the underlying mechanisms that shape our human experience and the complex interplay between our inner worlds and external realities. The challenge was, I couldn't quite articulate what I had learned. Psychedelics have this way of showing us life's magic, but putting that magic into words? Not so easy. Still, I was determined because the clarity I gained amazed me, and I knew it could benefit many others. I knew there was something profoundly simple within this complexity, and I was determined to learn how to articulate it just as simply as I saw it. That determination led me to the library, where I devoured every bit of knowledge I could find about the mind. And that's where I stumbled upon

Freud's theories, which aligned so closely with my own revelations that I was astounded by our parallel visions.

Freud observed a pattern of the psyche being compartmentalized into three distinct parts. He labeled them based on their developmental structure throughout our lives—those labels would be the ego, superego, and id.

That trio shapes how we think, act, and desire. Freud's breakdown of this trio provides a sensible explanation for the fluctuations in our thoughts and the depth to which they can travel or be stored. It can be tricky to catch our thoughts as they happen in the moment, making it tough for us to fully understand why we think and act the way we do. Freud's theory will help you grasp the rhythm and structure of your psyche, paving the way for a transformative grasp of your mind's true nature and its impact on your life's journey.

MEET EGO, SUPEREGO & ID

When most people think of someone with a big ego, they picture someone who's all about themselves or comes off as a bit arrogant. In reality, the ego is like a little compartment in your mind that tries to make sense of the world around you. The thing is, sometimes it can create conflicts between your thoughts and reality, especially when you're unaware of the deeper workings of your mind.

Picture your mind as this evolving system of thought and behavior. The id is that raw, primal part of you that just wants to fulfill basic needs and desires. Then there's the superego, which is like your internal rule book shaped by society and cultural upbringing, telling you what's right and wrong. And in the middle of all this is the ego, playing referee and trying to find a balance between what you want and what you should do according to the rules. It's like having three characters in your head, each with their own agenda, and the ego is the "executive" part of our mind, striving to keep the peace.

Initially, you might wonder how your id, superego, and ego are present within yourself, influencing your ways of thinking. Isn't it strange how difficult it can be to grasp and comprehend all the different facets of ourselves and how they work? Your mind, unlike your body, is incredibly malleable and multifaceted, far too complex to be understood by considering just one aspect of its multidimensional nature. Without realizing it, we often use a linear approach when trying to understand the complexities of the psyche. This tendency can lead to confusion when we attempt to impose structure or order on something as abstract as the mind. Imagine trying to use just one piece of a puzzle to figure out the whole picture; it's not so simple, as the mind, emotions, and inner workings of reality all come together. I find that taking a step back and looking at life from a broader perspective can bring clarity to these intricate concepts.

Envision your mind as a massive iceberg. What we see above the waterline is just the tip: your conscious thoughts, the ones you're aware of and actively think about. But beneath that surface lies this vast, hidden realm—the subconscious. It's where things get complex—housing everything from your deepest desires, your darkest fears, and memories that shape who you are.

CONSCIOUS LEVEL

SUBCONSCIOUS LEVEL

UNCONSCIOUS LEVEL

EGO

Within your psyche, the ego emerges as your conscious self, aiming to be rational based on the development and interplay of the id and superego—constantly balancing desires and reality, guiding daily decision-making.

SUPER EGO

Deeper within your psyche, the superego forms as your internal inner critic, influenced by external teachings and societal norms, shaping your values, ethics, and behavior.

ID

At the core, your id drives primal instincts, including pleasure-seeking urges like sex and impulses such as aggression, shaping your actions and choices.

THE RISE OF THE EGO

As big as that iceberg in the metaphor is, it barely scratches the surface of how vast and intricate our minds really are. This is why it can feel so tricky to recall specific memories, especially those heavy with trauma or negative emotions, often buried away where we believe they belong. They're submerged in the depths of our subconscious, like a hidden universe inside us, influencing our thoughts, emotions, and behaviors, even if we're not always aware of it. Yet, despite this vast reservoir of thoughts and emotions, we can go about our daily lives, seemingly unaffected. It's as if we're cruising along the surface, blissfully unaware of the depths beneath us, yet continuing forward despite the occasional rough patches we encounter along the way. This shows how our minds are incredibly complex yet adaptable, allowing us to function even with so much going on beneath the surface.

It's common for people to walk around masking their truth, unaware that their authentic selves have been buried deep within their subconscious. This heaviness weighs them down, and instead of acknowledging it, they tend to adjust to the weight, living their lives without realizing the magnitude of what's hidden inside them. It's like carrying a boulder in your chest, an emotional burden that shapes every aspect of your existence without your even noticing.

It's astonishing how we can navigate life, build a life, and share our existence with others while carrying such heavy burdens and hidden truths. This hidden weight not only adds more layers of falsehood but also intensifies the heaviness that defines our existence. It's an eye-opening realization, isn't it? How can our minds allow us to go through life unaware of deeply impact-ful and life-altering experiences, carrying hidden burdens that shape our existence without our conscious knowledge? Well, I've noticed how the ego can completely dominate and shape the narrative and perception of one's reality. It's like our ego becomes this silent guardian, swooping in when we're vul-nerable, shielding us from potential harm, pain, shame, or discomfort—shaping our reality to fit what we believe is safe or acceptable.

But here's the twist—I've also come to see the ego as more than just a protector. It actually becomes a character, shaped by our experiences, beliefs, and interactions with the world. Our superego, that internal moral compass, and our id, the primal force, they both play a part in shaping this ego character. How we think, how we behave to get what we want, how we see our-selves—it's all intertwined with this ego persona. And based on how the world responds to us, we adjust our script accordingly. Throughout our years we are unknowingly but constantly fine-tuning this character to navigate the grand stage of life. It's like we're constantly navigating this dance between who we are, who we think we should be, and how the world per-ceives us.

This is where we step into a cage, unknowingly becoming ensnared within our ego as it inadvertently takes center stage in shaping our perception. It's a delicate situation, where parts of ourselves remain unrecognized, yet they subtly govern our thoughts and actions. This extends beyond mere self-image; it influences our entire perspective of the world and our interac-tions with others.

As we go through life, the ego continuously evolves, shaped by each event and its consequences. Over time, the ego's perception of reality begins to dominate, filtering how we view the world. Our internal experiences—whether positive or negative—gradually shape the way we perceive and interpret our external reality.

INSIDE THE EGO: UNDERSTANDING YOUR IDENTITY

Within the study of psychology, experts have established the ego's core as the foundation of our identity and described its profound influence on our cognitive landscape. But let's break this down for the everyday person trying to understand their mind's inner workings.

The goal here is to grasp a clear understanding of the different versions of yourself that exist within your psyche—your id and superego—and how these aspects come together to form your ego persona. This process of unraveling your psyche piece by piece serves as the starting point to liberate yourself from a hidden cage, one that you may be completely unaware of.

Now, of course I don't know the details of your life story to pinpoint the moments that molded your ego, but I can still, without a doubt, tell you that everything you have become today is a reaction to experiences that impacted your emotions as well as the things you were exposed to. Your mind is still attracting, chasing, or running away from those experiences if you remain unaware of the emotions attached to these memories.

The subconscious mind holds incredible power and plays a crucial role in shaping our life stories. It guides our actions and reactions because our emotions and nervous system are closely tied to memories stored within it. This explains why many of our reactions are impulsive, sometimes leading to denial, dissociation, patterns of self-sabotage, or self-destructive behavior. Think of the brain as the central control system of a complex network, with the nervous system acting as an intricate web extending throughout your entire body. This structured web is designed to relay information, coordinating actions and responses. However, when emotions take hold, the dynamic shifts. Instead of the brain orchestrating from the depths of your mind, it becomes a slave to the body's immediate emotional experiences. Consider your nervous system as an elaborate matrix, each nerve transmitting the sensations and emotions that course through you. When emotions like fear, anxiety, or pain dominate, they hijack this network, making the brain focus on these immediate feelings rather than deeper, rational thoughts. This means that your reactions and decisions are driven more by the body's emotional state than by logical processes.

For instance, even if the discomfort is merely a memory, the nervous system can react as if the experience is happening in the present. The brain, in an attempt to avoid that emotional pain, will prioritize steering clear of anything that might bring up similar feelings again. This reflexive avoidance, whether triggered by big events or small moments, influences your decisions and can create a disconnect between what your mind knows logically and how your body reacts emotionally.

Instead of harmony being experienced within our mind and body, it's as if our bodies (emotions) are at war with our minds, and the ego assumes control, prolonging this conflict. This often leads us to avoid directly facing our feelings, causing us to disassociate from them. We struggle to define and understand these emotions, contributing to the ongoing conflict within ourselves.

On this battleground, the ego seizes control, embedding beliefs and justifications based on whatever emotions and thoughts trigger you. These beliefs then become a part of your character from that point forward. The ego creates a comfort zone or a safe haven around these beliefs, making it difficult to see beyond its walls. Emotional reactions act as the ammunition on this battlefield, overpowering our efforts to address the underlying issues, which adds another layer of complexity to the challenge of understanding ourselves.

For example, Freud came up with a concept called "penis envy." Basically, he believed that young girls at a certain stage start wishing they had a penis, not because they actually want one but because they see it as a symbol of power and respect, especially in a society that values masculinity. In psychology, this theory dives into the subconscious dynamics of psychosexual development; however, I perceive an even deeper layer to it.

Imagine a young girl, dismissed because of her gender and denied opportunities that are freely given to her male peers. Perhaps her mother tells her that certain ambitions or aspirations, like a career in engineering, aren't meant for girls, or discourages her from playing sports because "it's not ladylike." As she observes her brother or male peers receiving preferential treatment, a seed of resentment and anger begins to grow within her, though she may not consciously acknowledge these emotions. Let me be clear: she can absolutely feel these emotions as she experiences them, and she might even recognize her reactions. However, there's a profound difference between acknowledging and fully embracing the actual emotions versus just reacting to them. It's this fine line that forms the essence of this significant observation, showing how the perception of our egos takes over the experience of our individual reality.

In her young mind, the immediate logical conclusion emerges: if only she had been born with a penis, her life would be easier, fairer. This thought, born out of frustration and injustice, quietly plants a seed in her mind, shaping her perceptions and behaviors in small but important ways. Without her realizing it, these initial feelings of hurt and anger remain buried, influencing not just her perception of gender inequality but also her self-image and relationships with others. It's more than just wishing for the same opportunities as her male peers; she may unknowingly harbor resentment toward all males and even develop a sense of animosity as well as a lack of respect toward her mother.

The daughter might infer that if her mother believes there are things she cannot do or achieve simply because of her gender, the same must apply to her mother. This could lead her to subconsciously lose some respect for her mother as she starts to believe that being female comes with built-in limitations and a sense of unworthiness. As a result, the daughter's perception of her mother's capabilities and value could be shaped by the lessons she indirectly absorbs from her mother's views and restrictions.

Now, does she openly disrespect her mother? Not necessarily; maybe her superego won't let her. However, deep within, these feelings simmer. Her ego rationalizes this internal conflict by forming a subconscious aim to distance herself from her mother's views or to distrust her mother's guidance. This is where the ego rationalizes that having a penis would somehow solve her problems or grant her the respect and opportunities she feels she deserves. Instead of processing that she feels hurt and offended that her mother prioritizes societal standards over her passions and interests, she feels diminished, as if her mother believes her male peers and siblings are more capable than she is. This sense of being undervalued turns to disgust at her mother's narrow-mindedness and the audacity to impose such limiting beliefs on her. She feels deep resentment at the expectation to conform to her mother's way of life, knowing they are fundamentally different. Her hatred for a society that belittles women intensifies, leaving her overwhelmed by a torrent of emotions that surge through her so quickly she cannot consciously acknowledge each one.

This pivotal moment with her mother doesn't just affect her present emotions; it charts the course of her entire life. If she chooses to follow her mother's mindset, she might internalize a sense of weakness, subconsciously resenting herself for relinquishing control over her destiny. On the other hand, if she rebels, her life may be driven by a need to prove herself, sometimes leading her away from her true passions. This rebellion, fueled by a desire to show the world she can do anything a man can, can result in choices that aren't truly aligned with her core self. This single moment imprints on her identity, creating an ego persona that navigates life either through compliance or defiance, each with its own set of consequences. The emotional weight of this experience molds her worldview and influences her decisions, subtly steering her life's direction based on a single moment from a childhood confrontation.

As she ventures beyond her home and interacts with the wider world, she starts to notice how people's treatment of her is shaped by their perceptions and assumptions. This external feedback starts to intertwine with her own self-image, influencing how she sees herself and how she believes others view her. This dynamic creates a feedback loop where societal expectations and reactions significantly impact her self-perception and behavior. The way she is treated by others plays a crucial role in shaping her experiences and outlook on life, demonstrating how deeply external perceptions can affect our internal reality. Consequently, these external interactions slowly build a limiting framework around her mind, subtly tinting her reality and confining her sense of self within a constrained and often distorted perception.

This scenario is a common illustration of how our unacknowledged emotions influence our lives without our realizing it. These hidden emotions can lead us to make decisions aimed at comforting or dismissing the wounds we carry within, shaping our beliefs and actions in subtle yet impactful ways. Significantly, it's when our identity starts to take shape that we often lose touch with the natural flow of life. We begin to see everything through a particular lens, shaped by a specific narrative that's hard to break free from. Being stuck in this narrative confines us to a rigid way of thinking, hindering our growth and limiting our exploration.

When we respond from our ego, we often find ourselves caught in a cycle of justifying our reactions and defending our behavior. Instead of pausing to observe and understand the situation as it unfolds, we tend to react impulsively based on our immediate emotions. This reactive behavior reinforces our ego's persona, creating a self-justifying narrative that further shapes our identity and confines our understanding. The ego, driven by its need to protect and validate itself, blocks genuine insight and deeper awareness. By learning to navigate and express our emotions more consciously in the moment, we can break free from this limiting cycle, allowing for a more authentic and fluid experience of life and reducing the burden of ego-driven reactions.

Ah, if only personal transformation were as simple as flipping a switch. In reality, the journey to change our perception of ourselves and our lives is far more complex. Many struggle with this process, either because they don't fully grasp the need for change or because the ego obstructs their progress, making it feel like an uphill battle. Operating beneath our conscious awareness, the ego shapes our thoughts and behaviors in ways that can be hard to pinpoint. Even when we manage to track our thoughts, knowing how to navigate and act on these insights can be challenging. Embracing this path requires more than just a wish for change; it demands patience, introspection, and a keen understanding of the ego's subtle influence.

The challenge lies in understanding how our thoughts and emotions coexist and intertwine, as this seems to be at the core of our struggle to analyze situations as they arise and the experiences that shaped us. This is where diving into the relationship between your id and superego becomes incredibly enlightening.

UNCONSCIOUS FORCES: THE DOMINANCE OF ID AND SUPEREGO

Once upon a time, as a baby, you experienced life in its purest form, a whirlwind of emotions flowing freely. Frustration, anger, disappointment, desperation, happiness, joy, and love poured out of you without hesitation or restraint. This was the realm of your id, the unfiltered, selfish essence of your being. In this primal state, only your natural biological instincts mattered. You didn't pause to consider if your caretaker was tired or in pain; you communicated your needs with instinctual urgency, demanding immediate attention and fulfillment. It was a time when every desire, every need, was expressed with the raw authenticity of a newborn discovering the world. Of course you couldn't quite grasp an understanding of words yet, but you were definitely completely conscious of your own human existence and the patterns of people and things around you, enough to receive personal pleasure.

As you grew older, particularly between the ages of three to five, you began to be shaped in two distinct ways. First, you learned to tame your primal, instinctual behaviors. You know, the screaming to get your way, the temper tantrums, biting, throwing objects, and so on. And second, you adapted to coexist within our sophisticated construct of a society.

These very moments are the manipulation of your id and the birth of your superego, a time when your primitive nature was domesticated into a version that would fit into whatever environment you were born into. This is the perfect point to understand yourself from the superego's perspective, the very deepest part of you that lies beneath the surface of your self-image.

YOUR SUPEREGO

Your environment and the people who raised you play a significant role in shaping how you navigate the outside world. Many of us haven't actively chosen how we live our lives; we were born into circumstances or guided by life's unpredictable currents. The standards, emotions, beliefs, and values instilled by those around us all contribute to molding our mindset. These external influences often dictate our approach to life, setting the stage for how we respond to challenges and opportunities.

Some aspects of your behavior and habits may feel normal solely because of what you were taught—intentionally or circumstantially. These teachings form the foundation of how you perceive yourself and engage with your reality. This may already be very obvious to you, but it's also very common to miss the connection between your experiences and your behavior. It often takes comparing ourselves to others to recognize our own ways of thinking or being. In social settings like school or outside activities, we may start to notice these differences, yet it can still be challenging to truly grasp our own behavior. We're often too immersed in being ourselves to pay close attention to our own actions and thoughts.

Our thoughts are constantly racing, often between different perspectives. This phenomenon is facilitated by our superego acting as a mediator between the id and the external world. This complex compartmentalization leads to a separation between who we present to the world and our internal reality. This division can sometimes create a distortion in understanding our true selves, as the external and internal worlds start to diverge. Society often encourages us to prioritize the version of ourselves that is more socially acceptable, whether that means embracing certain aspects or disconnecting from certain aspects. This internal-external divide often results in two distinct worlds in our life: the world of our thoughts and the world of our actions. These parallel realities often feel distant from each other because capturing all our unfiltered thoughts can be incredibly challenging.

Let's revisit the earlier example of the girl grappling with "penis envy." Picture a scenario where she's all grown up and now finds herself in a conversation with her female friend. That conversation years ago with her mother still sits inside of her, dictating the sway of her thoughts. So when her friend expresses her passion for becoming a homemaker, she feels a surge of internal conflict. Outwardly, she tries to be supportive, but deep inside, subconscious judgment and resentment surface. She chooses to be supportive to her friend but ends up feeling a bit of disrespect for her, subtly shifting how she views her. On the surface, being a supportive friend is important to her, so she ignores these thoughts, especially because those other thoughts do not reflect well on her behalf.

This inner conflict stems from her superego dictating how she should think and behave to align with societal expectations, while old memories and emotions contradict this. Her super-ego, aiming to present an acceptable and likable version of herself, overrides her true feelings. This version is the one she shows to the world, and over time, she begins to believe that this is her only self. Those buried thoughts and emotions seem irrelevant, even nonexistent, because she is so focused on maintaining the image others expect. As a result, the genuine parts of her, those connected to deeper subconscious thoughts, are suppressed. She believes this curated self is her true iden-tity, pushing aside any conflicting feelings or memories and overshadowing the more complex and authentic parts of her personality. Without even realizing it, she has let her superego mask her true self, leading her to live a life that aligns more with external expectations than with her inner reality.

As we navigate through life, our thoughts and actions often follow patterns dictated by our subconscious mindset. This becomes particularly complex when dealing with trauma or painful experiences. Internally, we grapple with processing our true thoughts and emotions, while externally, we conform to societal norms. This creates a third reality, where the superego crafts a distorted version of ourselves—a persona shaped by who we need to be to coexist within society. This version isn't just a facade; it's reinforced by the reactions and treatment we receive based on this persona, leading us to believe in it as our true self. Imagine how much of our lives, from major decisions to everyday interactions, are influenced by this mindset. This third reality becomes dominant, overshadowing our authen-tic self and shaping our entire existence. Consequently, our conscious self begins to prioritize this crafted aspect of our mind, blurring the lines between who we truly are and who we think we need to be. This conflict highlights the importance of understanding the id.

YOUR ID

Terms like "primal," "natural," and "instinctual" come up time and time again when discussing the id. That's because these words form the very core of our being, rooted in our mammalian nature. Food, shelter, and sex—these primal needs remind us of who we truly are beneath the layers of civilization and advancement. Think about it—our primal instincts, embodied in the id, are the raw, unfiltered impulses that stem from our basic needs and desires. They serve as a tether to our animalistic essence, constantly reminding us that deep down, we're simply another species in the grand scheme of life.

It may sound silly, but our first layer of an ego death is simply remembering that we are human. For a moment, forget about your job, your hobbies, your religion, and even the color of your skin. You are first and foremost a human experiencing modern life. You may be too fixated on the details of your life, so much that the thought of who you are doesn't exactly cross your mind. This is why many people experimenting with altered states using psychedelics or even marijuana often focus intensely on sensations like their heartbeat or the functionality of their hands. Heightened awareness can highlight how we often go through life without truly being aware of our own existence.

As humans, we stand out not just for our intelligence but also for our insatiable quest for pleasure, comfort, and love. While other species also follow societal norms or behavioral guidelines, we're driven by a deep desire to experience joy, seek solace, and forge meaningful connections—both within ourselves and in the world around us. In the animal kingdom, these pursuits might seem like luxuries, but for us, they seem to be the driving forces behind our advancement.

It's fascinating to consider that the foundation of our progress and innovation stems from the challenges and inconveniences that come with our mammalian nature. Despite our evolution into sophisticated beings, we're still fundamentally driven by instincts rooted in our mammalian origins.

Your id represents your primal core of emotions. Remember, during infancy your emotions were expressed exactly as they were felt, without any consideration for others or remorse— the primal version of you knew to express your truth no matter what. However, as we mature, we learn to manage our emotions, becoming more aware of their impact on those around us and how these interactions, in turn, affect our own emotional state. Our compartmentalized brains start to choose carefully which emotions to experience and express. This understanding serves as a gateway to dive deeper into our connection or disconnection with our emotional selves.

THE ID'S LANGUAGE IN THE SUPEREGO'S WORLD

As we navigate the complexities of the external world, societal norms often pressure us to temper, compress, and even suppress the untamed language of emotions. We're conditioned to believe that openly expressing our emotions is somehow uncivilized, undesirable, or even inconvenient. Though adapting to social norms can sometimes be practical, it often comes at the cost of losing touch with our true emotional depth. This disconnection has far-reaching consequences, impacting our internal well-being and holistic health. It also marks the transition where our emotions transform from being our first language to becoming our burdens.

Actually, it's during the transition into young adulthood that emotions can start feeling burdensome. Puberty is far more than just a change between developmental stages; it's an intense shift in emotion, energy, and mentality, all in preparation for procreation—a fundamental instinct shared by all species.

The hormonal shifts we experience within the mind and body may feel reminiscent of the emotional whirlwind encountered in infancy—equally intense but now with a heightened sense of awareness. These powerful emotions, especially those tied to sexuality, flow naturally with our primal instincts. However, understanding and managing these emotions can be tricky, particularly given the complexities of sexuality and the unspoken societal norms surrounding it. Even with the superego's influence shaping our psyche, these hormonal shifts bring back familiar and powerful feelings that don't always align with the constructed reality of the superego. The emotions tied to sexuality and the hormonal changes during menstruation carry a significant intensity that often disrupts everyday routines and mindsets.

What's particularly dangerous is how sexuality, embedded so deeply within our biology, inevitably creates another compartmentalized version of ourselves. This version often remains far separated from the others, as our biological impulses do not always align with the superego's constructed reality. The superego acts as a protective wall around these instinctual experiences, especially within our social constructs. While this is understandable as we coexist within our sophisticated society, it doesn't alter our mental and emotional impulses. Instead, we further suppress our energy and emotions under the superego's influence, adding yet another layer to our ego persona.

This compartmentalization results in distinct versions of ourselves, each operating separately and creating a fragmented self-perception. Our intimate thoughts and profound emotions, though hidden, continue to influence our thoughts and actions subtly. It's like having a hidden chamber in your psyche where these primal urges and intense emotions reside. While we may dismiss these aspects of ourselves, they continue to shape our experiences and behaviors in ways we may not fully comprehend. By recognizing this, we can begin to understand the dynamics of our compartmentalized minds and how they impact our overall sense of self.

These layers of ego persona formation become more ingrained as we move into adulthood, making it increasingly challenging to fully understand ourselves or navigate our own thought processes. We are not just learning to manage emotions; we are also grappling with the following:

+ Adapting to social expectations
+ Taming our primal urges
+ Perceiving life through the lens of beliefs adapted from our upbringing
+ Balancing how we want to be viewed with how we perceive ourselves

✦ Internally and externally reacting to emotionally impactful experiences
✦ Protecting ourselves from resurfacing pain
✦ Concealing aggression and sexual desires to maintain civility

Each of these layers, which form before we even begin to understand the immense power our minds hold, adds complexity to our psyche, fragmenting our sense of self and reality. It's no wonder that our thought processes can feel overwhelming and disjointed.

On top of all of that, our ego persona carries the emotional intelligence and maturity we've adapted through life's shifts and changes, shaping how we navigate the journey ahead. The ego filters our personal realities, influencing our interpretations and responses, ultimately molding us into the individuals we are today.

All of this complexity creates a multilayered persona before we even learn who we truly are. However, there is a silver lining: recognizing the incredible power our minds hold is a hidden gem. The fact that our minds can function as a unified entity within one body, while also being divided and compartmentalized, shows the extraordinary capabilities we possess. This ability to carry specific awareness and adapt it to our lives, despite the layers and compartments, is proof of the mind's true magic.

But the real beauty lies in how our brains operate beneath the surface. Our thoughts, emotions, and behaviors are not random; they follow specific patterns that our minds have learned over time. These patterns are shaped by neural pathways—connections in our brain that form when we repeat certain actions, thoughts, or emotions. Imagine these pathways as well-worn trails in a forest. The more we think or behave in a certain way, the more deeply entrenched these trails become, making it easier for our brain to travel the same route again and again.

Initially, these pathways develop as we move through life, learning from our experiences and adjusting to our surroundings. But here's the fascinating part: just as these pathways are created, they can also be reshaped. With awareness and intention, you can consciously create new pathways, changing the patterns that no longer serve you. By doing this, you're not just breaking old habits or healing from past traumas—you're rewiring your brain, giving yourself the power to transform your thoughts, emotions, and experiences. This isn't just mental; it's physical. Your brain is literally changing.

Recognizing the incredible power and depth of our minds is just the beginning. The true magic lies in the realization that we have the power to choose how to use our minds and live our lives. Despite the compartmentalized nature of our thoughts and emotions, which can often make us feel as though we're merely continuing the life we've been led into, we hold the potential to reclaim our narrative.

As we navigate the twists and turns of our unique paths, there comes a moment for many of us when the persona we've crafted starts to feel overwhelming and constricting. It's as if we're suffocating under the weight of a self that no longer fits. We become acutely aware of a profound disconnection from the essence of who we truly are, feeling lost and disoriented by the layers of identity that have been shaped and reshaped by external influences. This sense of being out of touch with our deeper selves can be disheartening, leaving us questioning the very core of our existence and our true purpose in life. An ego death represents a powerful process of shedding these imposed layers and rediscovering our genuine selves, free from the filters and masks we've adopted. It reconnects us with the depths of our being so we can embrace a sense of authenticity that transcends the roles we've been molded into over time.

BEYOND THE EGO

As our minds become preoccupied with managing the various compartments of our psyche—each layer shaped by societal expectations and personal survival—the ego becomes intricately entwined with our sense of self, overshadowing our deeper truth. We start to view ourselves solely as human beings navigating a complex social landscape, rather than recognizing that we are also spiritual beings with a profound connection to something greater. This keeps us from fully grasping the larger, more meaningful aspects of our existence, as we remain absorbed in the surface-level struggles and achievements of our daily lives.

Navigating the maze of our compartmentalized minds often means losing touch with the profound interconnectedness of our being. In the midst of managing all these layers, we might forget that we are not just a collection of fragments but a harmonious blend of body, mind, and spirit.

To help clarify this, I've included a simple graph. It's meant to give you a clearer view of how our psyche relates to these layers—mind, body, and spirit—showing how they interact and influence each other. This visual aims to offer a new perspective on our multidimensional nature and the unity that ties us all together.

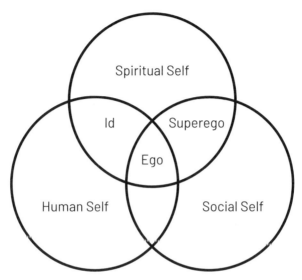

The aim of the ego death experience is to integrate this self-knowledge into a unified human experience.

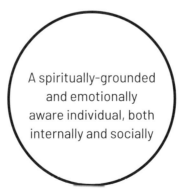

At its core, life is simple—it's our individual journeys that make it feel complicated. This is where my personal discovery, the

1-3-2 method, comes into play. This method is designed to enhance clarity and fluidity in navigating your state of mind to help you journey through life gracefully and authentically. But before diving into the 1-3-2 method, it's essential to grasp the workings of perception, which is further refined by your unique personality. This paves the way for unraveling each layer of yourself during the ego death process—leading you to rediscover the core of your truth.

CHAPTER 2

PERSONALITY PERCEPTION

Understanding personality perception isn't necessarily rocket science; instead, it's seen as complex because it introduces an additional layer to our understanding of our reality. And on the journey toward an ego death, a big goal is to dismantle all things blocking the higher self and life's bigger picture.

Your personality presents a significant obstacle in bridging the gap between you and your fullest and highest potential. How? Well, your personality is as inevitable as your psyche; it's fundamental to the way you experience life through your own eyes. Your personality is like a role you're born to play in life, shaping not just how you perceive but also how you interact with the world. This familiarity with your role can make it incredibly challenging to see beyond it, as it becomes a microcosm—your exclusive lens for understanding reality. Your ego constantly reinforces and justifies these perceptions, solidifying your view of the world through the filter of your personality.

It's easy to get lost in this familiar space, but it's also crucial to recognize that there's more to life than just our immediate perceptions. While getting a handle on our personalities might feel easier than diving into our psyche's complexities, it's a whole new challenge to shift how we see our experiences throughout our lives.

This part of the journey isn't about disregarding your personality nor about losing yourself; who you are at your core is your birthright. Rather, it's about uncovering another layer that hides the precious gem within you, allowing you to grow and expand your dimensions of self-existence.

Getting to know different parts of yourself is like adjusting a camera lens, zooming in or out to see the finer details. Think of it like this: your psyche is like the canvas of your reality, providing the foundational materials for your life's story. Meanwhile, your personality is like the filter, adding depth and color to how you interpret and move through this reality. By breaking down these dimensions of self piece by piece, you're essentially priming yourself for a gradual ego death process. It's like laying the groundwork for understanding yourself before diving into deeper introspection, whether through psychedelics or other methods. As you grasp the dynamics of your role in shaping your experiences, you gain insight into how your choices and perceptions steer the course of your life's journey.

DEFAULT SETTINGS: THE ROLE OF PERSONALITY IN DAILY LIVING

Life is filled with daily challenges, victories, and everything in between. In the midst of our busy schedules and constant demands, it can be challenging to step back and view life as a continuous journey. We become engrossed in the immediacy of our experiences, focusing on what life seems to throw our way, without always pausing to reflect on the broader path we're traveling.

As you've already learned, at the core of our being, emotions silently guide us, laying the foundation for the journey we tread. They shape our perceptions, decisions, and ultimately, the path we unknowingly carve for ourselves.

While on the surface, it's our personalities that take the lead, shaping how we navigate along this carved path. Outside of our emotional realm, we operate on a smaller scale, focusing on our day-to-day lives based on our personalities—our jobs, how we spend our time, how we present ourselves, and what captures our attention each day. This dynamic is crucial because, well, it's where most of our focus lies, and in life, attention is like a currency—it draws things in and out of our lives.

You've likely come across this phrase: "the law of attraction." Here's the deal: many of us are either drawing things toward us or pushing them away without even realizing it, and much of this is due to our default settings, shaped by the roles we play through our egos and personalities.

PERSONA AND PERSONALITY: EXPLORING YOUR CHARACTER ARCHETYPE

Taking the time to observe and understand your personality is like unlocking the next level of self-perception. On this level you'll be turning on a brighter light in the room of self-awareness, illuminating not just yourself but also the narratives of your life. This newfound clarity serves as a guiding light as we explore even deeper layers of our identity, shedding light on the mechanisms of our default settings.

As you dive into the exploration of your personality and seek to understand yourself on a deeper level, the Myers-Briggs Type Indicator (MBTI) becomes an invaluable tool. Developed by Katherine Cook Briggs and her daughter, Isabel Briggs Myers, this chart is based on Carl Jung's theory of psychological types, offering a structured framework to categorize and understand human personalities. It's like stepping into the role of a spectator, analyzing the details of your own character. Take your time to thoroughly assess who you believe you are, examining your preferences, tendencies, and behaviors. For a more detailed evaluation, consider taking a free online test that uses the Myers-Briggs system.

In essence, this straightforward framework acts as a guide to understanding both your personal characteristics and the role you play in the grand narrative of life.

THE FOUR MBTI PREFERENCE PAIRS

EXTRAVERSION	INTROVERSION

Opposite ways to direct and receive energy

SENSING	INTUITION

Opposite ways to take in information

THINKING	FEELING

Opposite ways to decide and come to conclusions

JUDGING	PERCEIVING

Opposite ways to approach the outside world

Energizing Focus: Are You Extraverted or Introverted?

Consider how you recharge and express your energy. Are you someone who thrives in social settings, finding energy in interactions and external activities (extraversion)? Or do you feel more invigorated and centered in quieter, reflective moments, drawing energy from your inner thoughts and feelings (introversion)?

Learning Style: Observational or Imaginative?

Think about how you prefer to gather information and make sense of the world. Do you rely heavily on tangible, concrete data from your senses and immediate environment (sensing)? Or do you often trust your instincts, insights, and internal patterns, seeking meaning beyond what's directly observable (intuition)?

Decision-Making Style: Logic or Emotion?

Reflect on how you process and evaluate information to make decisions. Do you prioritize objective analysis, logic, and reason, aiming to be fair and practical in your decision-making or choices (thinking)? Or do you tend to weigh decisions based on personal values, emotions, and empathy, valuing harmony and emotional resonance (feeling)?

Problem-Solving Mode: Structured or Flexible?

Consider how you navigate plans, schedules, and life's uncertainties. Are you someone who prefers structure, organization, and predictability, finding comfort in plans and routines (judging)? Or do you embrace spontaneity, adaptability, and open-mindedness, enjoying the freedom to explore new possibilities and adapt as situations unfold (perceiving)?

By diving into these dimensions, you unlock insights into your distinctive preferences and habits, leading to a richer comprehension of the character you play in life's grand narrative. Your personality archetype serves as the scriptwriter, shaping your actions and interactions within the stage set by your psyche. This perspective offers a higher vantage point, allowing you to envision your life as a captivating story, with your character at the forefront, navigating through the plotlines dictated by your unique traits and tendencies.

PERSONALITY TYPE CHART

	INTROVERT	INTROVERT	EXTRAVERT	EXTRAVERT	
THINKING	**ISTJ** Practical and fact minded; very reliable	**INTJ** Imaginative and strategic; have a plan for everything	**ESTJ** Excellent administrators; unsurpassed at managing people	**ENTJ** Bold, imaginative; always finding a way or making one	**JUDGING**
THINKING	**ISTP** Bold and practical experimenters; masters of all kinds of tools	**INTP** Innovative inventors with an unquenchable thirst for knowledge	**ESTP** Smart, energetic, perceptive; enjoy living on the edge	**ENTP** Smart and curious; cannot resist an intellectual challenge	**PERCEIVING**
FEELING	**ISFJ** Very dedicated and protective; always ready to defend their loved ones	**INFJ** Quiet and mystical yet inspiring; tireless idealists	**ESFJ** Extraordinarily caring, social, popular, and always eager to help	**ENFJ** Charismatic and inspiring leaders; able to mesmerize their listeners	**JUDGING**
FEELING	**ISFP** Flexible and charming artists; always ready to explore and experience something new	**INFP** Poetic, kind, and altruistic; always eager to help a good cause	**ESFP** Spontaneous, energetic, and enthusiastic entertainers; never boring	**ENFP** Enthusiastic, creative free spirits who can always find a reason to smile	**PERCEIVING**
	SENSING	INTUITIVE	SENSING	INTUITIVE	

Source: Myers & Briggs Foundation

PERSONALITY'S INFLUENCE ON LIFE'S PATH

Consider the intriguing idea of there being 16 archetypes, representing the diverse variations in how people think, feel, and perceive the world. With over a billion individuals on Earth, it's fascinating how only 16 fundamental types of personalities may exist. This perspective encourages us to reflect deeply on the role of our default settings—our ingrained personality traits that govern our thoughts, actions, and responses, intertwined with the backdrop of our life circumstances.

Our default settings operate much like being lost in a dream where you're immersed in a scene, without questioning how you arrived there. We're so engrossed in playing our character that we rarely question the why or how of it all. It's almost trippy when you think about it—our internal world, our psyche, shaping our external reality without us even realizing it.

Have you ever noticed how elusive it is to truly understand ourselves without the aid of personality charts or tests? It's fascinating how we require external guidance to perceive ourselves from a higher perspective. Without this insight, we tend to operate on autopilot, with our actions and experiences passing by unnoticed, driven by the familiar patterns ingrained within us. We live each day as we've been crafted to, following the paths set by our personalities. It's like we've been cast in a role we can't easily step out of; we wake up each day embodying the same character, playing out our unique storyline as if programmed to do so.

We're deeply immersed in experiencing our behaviors rather than observing them. Our personalities shape our view of reality so intensely that it can be hard to naturally see beyond our own perspectives. This highlights the potency and importance of perception in our human journeys, revealing how easily we overlook ourselves when our focus lies elsewhere. The pivotal question then becomes: Where is our perception truly focused, and what might we be missing because of this focused lens?

When we dive deeper into our background stories and how they shape our psyches, then further contemplate how our personalities steer this very specific narrative, it leads us to question the concept of destiny: Why are we who we are, existing within the complexity of our lives?

It's almost as if our personalities, our unique archetypes, are more than just our preferences and behaviors; personality seems to also be about the unique role of our archetypes. They also contribute our storyline to the larger narrative of life.

Each event, each pain, each triumph, seems to have a purpose, directing us exactly where we were meant to be. Strangely, these experiences may also direct the narrative of another's life. The way events and personalities interact really encourages us to think deeply and look beyond our day-to-day lives. While our daily routines often capture our attention, they are just fragments of our larger narrative. Our story began unfolding from the time we entered this world, and the present moment invites us to reflect on the journey that has shaped us into who we are right now. Who we are now determines how we continuously experience our reality and the paths that we continue to carve.

So, take a moment to reflect on your journey. Can you recognize your character within this captivating narrative of existence? As you navigate through the scenes and chapters of your life, pause to consider the impact of your personality, your choices, and your interactions with others. You're not merely drifting through each day; you're actively shaping a narrative. Every thought, action, and decision you make contributes to the plot. Your role is significant, and your story is ongoing.

Just like in any captivating story or film, our lives are filled with an ensemble cast of characters, each playing their unique roles in various narratives. We're not just the protagonists of our own stories; we're also supporting characters, rivals, allies, and antagonists in the tales of others. Each of us has a purpose within the larger plot, contributing to the richness and depth of the overarching storyline. Our lives blend together to create a kaleidoscope of experiences, emotions, and lessons.

Yet, seeing the bigger picture can be tough when we're dealing with our personal experiences. When we're in the thick of our experiences, every detail, internal or external, adds layers of complexity that can be overwhelming. But if we could step back, just for a moment, and view these experiences from a broader perspective, we might find clarity amidst the chaos.

Imagine watching a movie where you, as the observer, can clearly see what the character should or should not do. As you're comfortably watching from your home, you're cringing or feeling desperate for the character to see things clearly because it seems so obvious to you. You understand that character's motivations and experiences, yet you also have a certain expectation or hope for how the story should unfold.

However, for the character immersed in the emotions of that scene, their perception is limited to how they feel. As the tense scene unfolds, the character finds themself at a crossroads, torn between two crucial choices that will determine their fate. They're engulfed in a whirlwind of emotions—fear, doubt, and a glimmer of hope. From the outside, it's evident what the best course of action would be, but for the character, the weight of their past experiences, regrets, and aspirations clouds their judgment. As the clock ticks, you're on the edge of your seat, rooting for the character to break free from their limitations and make the right choice. But alas, the character's perception remains locked within their personal narrative, unable to fully grasp the bigger picture that you, the observer, see so clearly.

Similarly, we are simply characters in our own stories, deeply immersed in the emotions and patterns woven by the ego and subconscious. These elements dictate our decisions and responses, anchoring us in our roles without our realizing the power to alter our narrative. Life seems straightforward when we're observing. It's the weight of our journeys that turns it into a maze-like experience—where the mind and body navigate through a labyrinth of emotions, memories, and beliefs.

What if you could shift your perspective, viewing your life as a detached observer? Imagine the clarity and insight that could bring, seeing beyond the immediate emotions and experiences that often weigh you down. This shift allows you to seize control of your life's narrative, becoming the architect of your own story and infusing it with intentionality to create a storyline that truly resonates with and impresses you.

In our journeys through life, we've weathered countless storms, often feeling like we've had little control over our circumstances. It's almost as if we've become accustomed to this lack of control, so much so that when the tides shift and suddenly, we have the power to steer our own narrative, it can be overwhelming to realize that the story is now in our hands, to recognize and accept this newfound control.

Take a moment to let this sink in—within the spectrum of the 16 archetypes, there are 15 other sets of perceptions and characteristics waiting to be explored (see page 49). This means that by identifying with just one, we are potentially limiting ourselves. Imagine the possibilities when you realize that, after an ego death, you can embody any of these archetypes. Different situations and scenarios often require different mindsets and characteristics, and recognizing this can empower you to adapt and thrive in any circumstance. You have the freedom to shape your reality and the ability to tap into the full range of human potential.

THE INTERPLAY OF INNER AND OUTER WORLDS: PSYCHE VS. PERSONALITY

Although these archetypes represent the roles we identify with, they don't define our entire existence. These roles reflect how we tend to think and act, shaping the theme of our life's story. However, the depth of your character and the unique way you navigate your life are sculpted by your psyche. It's the backdrop of your experiences and inner world that truly defines your reality, influencing how you play your role. Remember, you're far more complex and multifaceted than any single label or role.

From the moment you are born through every stage of life, your reality is built upon the foundation laid by your upbringing. Your psyche, composed of the id, ego, and superego, is continuously shaped by the experiences you go through, even if you don't actively notice it. It's shaped by what you were exposed to or shielded from, the treatment you received, the environments you grew up in, and the standards of living that framed your early years. This foundation extends deeply into your emotional well-being, life standards, and even your worldview, shaping the lens through which you perceive the world around you.

As you take charge of your life, you inevitably find yourself living within the standards and beliefs that have shaped you so far. Each event, emotion, and encounter becomes a pivotal part of your unique storyline, contributing to your perception and understanding of reality.

Think of your personality as the unique filter through which you experience your life's movie. Just like how each scene in a film is perceived differently depending on the camera angle, lighting, and setting, your personality adds depth and color to your experiences. And just like no two movies are exactly alike, no two people with the same personality type will experience life in the exact same way.

For example, imagine two INFP personality types who work together. On the surface, they might appear very similar, sharing the same cognitive functions and values. However, a deeper look into their backgrounds reveals stark differences that shape their perceptions and realities uniquely.

Let's say that one INFP grew up in the shadow of loss and responsibility. Picture a child who, at a tender age, faced the devastating pain of losing a parent. This trauma colored every aspect of their existence. With the remaining parent often absent due to the burden of providing for the family, this young INFP had to step into adult roles prematurely. They became not just a sibling but a caretaker, protector, and source of stability for their younger siblings. This experience shaped their reality into one where fragility and resilience were everyday norms.

Now, shift your focus to the other INFP, who carried the heavy secret of childhood abuse. This individual learned early about the darkness that can lurk behind closed doors. Unable to process the complexity of their trauma, they buried it deep within, shrouded in shame and confusion. Their reality became a narrative of fear, silence, and a relentless quest to maintain an illusion of normalcy. This burden of secrecy etched a unique lens through which they viewed the world, one colored by mistrust, self-doubt, and a longing for safety.

These contrasting narratives vividly illustrate how our backgrounds shape our realities. Our personalities then transform into the lenses through which we experience and interpret these storylines. However, our psyches, deeply intertwined with our emotions, add another layer to our perception of life.

Consider the first INFP, whose journey through loss and responsibility cultivated a deep empathy for others' pain and struggles, making them compassionate and caring. Their resilience allowed them to bear the emotional weight of their responsibilities. Yet, their psyche's relentless focus on caring for others left little room for self-reflection or personal care. This emotional landscape, defined by self-sacrifice and familial duty, often led to a disconnection from their own emotions. Their role as a caretaker, in which emotional neglect was common, permeated all areas of their life. This led them to feel defeated and isolated, which likely affected their relationships by attracting those who depended on them or reinforced their caregiver role. This lens of self-sacrifice made emotional detachment feel strangely comfortable, revealing a deeper dimension of their character in another perception of reality.

Conversely, the second INFP's empathetic nature, combined with their experience of abuse, led them to a quest for self-understanding and healing. Their idealism and creativity offered refuge from harsh realities. However, their psyche grappled with the realization that life is filled with hidden scars and unspoken truths. This realization, though not consciously acknowledged, subtly shaped their perception of human connections, keeping the depth of their inner world a mystery to themselves and those closest to them. Their lingering feelings of pain and fear seeped into their relationships, where their self-image reflected the hidden scars they carried, dictating their actions and interactions with others. This likely left them feeling uninspired by their own identity, struggling with a sense of emptiness and disconnection. Their reality became a labyrinth of secrets and suppressed emotions, a mask of normalcy while they grappled to reconcile their past with their present.

The personality is the external self, the visible face we show to others, while the psyche is the internal self, often hidden from both the world and even ourselves. These are two distinct worlds that coexist within us, each influencing our lives in different ways.

WHAT HAPPENS WHEN OUR INNER WORLD CONFLICTS WITH OUR OUTER PERSONA?

This dynamic between the inner world and the outer persona creates a version of reality that feels undeniably normal to us. These INFPs don't see themselves as broken or needing to be fixed; they see their experiences as their truths, shaping how they view the world. We often become so used to our emotional realities that we fail to see beyond them, trapped within the confines of our inner worlds.

Our unique emotional experiences steer our lives, influencing where our minds are willing to go or not go. It's these small details, accumulated over time, that turn our life experiences into individualistic, intricate journeys—much like the unique combinations of a Rubik's Cube.

Imagine starting life as a solved Rubik's Cube, with all the colors perfectly aligned, representing the shared beginnings we all have as humans with a soul, mind, and heart. As we navigate through life, each twist and turn—the experiences we encounter, the challenges we face, and the lessons we learn—rearranges the cube's colors in unique patterns. With every event, our perspectives shift, and our views of reality become distinctly our own.

Now, envision everyone walking around with their own Rubik's Cube, each one a complex, personalized mosaic of their life's journey. While we might glance at others' cubes, we're often deeply engrossed in our own, believing our combination to be the definitive view of life. In reality, what feels normal and all-encompassing to us is just one of countless unique configurations, each shaped by the details of our personal experiences.

Our personas—the archetypes we identify with—are versions of ourselves that are often difficult for us to see clearly. We can't see ourselves the way others do because we are too immersed in our internal world. Take the INFP who lost a parent, for example. They project a persona of compassion and care, which is how their siblings and friends experience them. However, this INFP doesn't get to experience this version of themself the way others do. Instead, they are shaped by their own emotional reality—feelings of neglect and loneliness due to not receiving the same love and compassion they give to others. This creates a conflict, as their persona is at odds with their lived experience. However, it's not that these aspects are truly in conflict—it's about perception. While others experience what you project, you only experience how you feel.

Our perception is just one part of a much larger and more complex picture. Only by acknowledging this can we begin to see the entirety of our character and move towards a more comprehensive self-awareness.

Your journey through ego death is like solving the puzzle of a Rubik's Cube, aligning all the pieces back to their original form. This process is not just about achieving balance, but also about recognizing how your current perception impacts your personal life, how you treat yourself, and the life you lead.

One of the crucial layers of ego death is seeing yourself, your character, in a different light and learning to steer your life's direction from that newfound understanding.

It's about aligning all the dimensions of your being—mind, heart, and soul—into a harmonious whole. Imagine the profound peace of having your inner colors harmonize, reflecting the true essence of who you are, with all dimensions of you existing harmoniously in the present moment. It's a beautiful process of rediscovery, where you see yourself clearly and connect deeply with the essence of your being. By aligning your perception back to the center of your existence and reality, you can see the full picture of who you are and the potential you hold. This broader view allows you to connect deeply with your true self and understand the essence of your being.

Essentially, our life experiences mold our psyches, deeply influencing the life we manifest and the reality we construct. An ego death reveals just how intricate and layered our minds and lives have become, showing that to truly understand ourselves, we must journey through the perception of our personality and the reality built by our psyche. Our perception, while vast in potential, is often tethered to the limitations of our psyches. Before experiencing an ego death, we may not fully utilize the potential of our characters or lives because our abilities are usually constrained by these limitations. The journey of self-awareness shows us how we tend to restrict ourselves to a narrow view of life, overlooking the vastness of reality that exists beyond our immediate experiences.

Embracing these insights is important for an ego death transformation, opening the door to a perspective beyond your character and initiating the unraveling of your ego. You have the power to change anything and everything about your character and the role you play in life. By cultivating this self-awareness, you can steer your life with intention, rather than simply drifting along on autopilot—letting your ego, subconscious patterns, and beliefs dictate your story.

As you reflect on these words, consider your own personal experiences and upbringing. How have they shaped the lens through which you view the world? There's a distinct difference between the character we present to the world and the version of ourselves we are when it's just us, alone with our thoughts. Behind closed doors, in those moments of solitude, we find ourselves in raw authenticity. How we spend that time and the emotions it evokes reveal the truest versions of ourselves— our personal perceptions untainted by external influences. When there's nothing and no one else to alter or influence our experience, our view of life emerges in its purest form, showcasing the unique differences that make us who we are. Recognizing this distinction allows us to see how the persona we project outwardly might differ from the deeply personal, internal reality we experience.

PERSONAL PERCEPTION

Each person inhabits their own remote island, complete with unique customs and a language of their own. Despite the desire to explore and connect, they remain stranded on their island, unable to venture to others' shores and truly understand life from their perspective. And even though we're all in a similar predicament of being stranded on our individual islands, our lenses and perceptions in life often divert our attention from realizing that we're on separate islands in the first place. The true challenge isn't just reaching others' islands but first recognizing the contours and limitations of our own; this sparks the journey to understanding the power of personal perception.

When you interact with someone else's reality, whether briefly or significantly, understanding each other completely becomes a challenge. Everyone you encounter becomes a supporting character in your story, their actions and words interpreted through your personal thoughts and beliefs. Simultaneously, you are just a character in their story, viewed through their own distinct lens.

Our observations about others typically merge their surface-level characteristics with our own projections influenced by our self-perception and past experiences. It's a subconscious process we engage in constantly, filtering the world through the lenses of our unique realities.

While we may strive to understand others and be understood, the complexities of individual experiences and perspectives often make it challenging to achieve true comprehension of one another. True comprehension would require knowing every single detail and event in someone's life—something impossible for anyone other than that individual. The nature of reality is truly mind-bending. It reveals how our distinct experiences, shaped by our minds and personalities, sculpt the worlds we perceive.

Taking a closer look at the role you play in your life story and recognizing how your narrative unfolds can be incredibly enlightening. It opens the door to a wider range of perceptions, allowing you to gain deeper insights into yourself and the world around you. The more perspectives you explore, the more aligned and prepared you become for a profound shift in consciousness.

I mention all of this to highlight the operation of your reality, as viewing this perspective can prompt you to question the true nature of reality itself. Looking back throughout my own journey, I realize that everything and nothing is real—it's all simply an experience unfolding, each individual playing their leading role, all interconnected and weaving into a larger, cohesive picture that we often overlook as we get caught up in our own narratives.

Many people become so immersed in their roles that they become blinded by them. Recognizing that life holds more than just these roles can be a liberating realization. When the layer of personal perception unravels during your moments of ego death, this can lead to a simpler and more peaceful navigation of life as you realize the expansiveness of your mind beyond its predefined role.

CHAPTER 3

✳ ☽ ✳

REALITY

When you hear the word "reality," what's the first image that pops into your mind? Is it a collage of personal experiences, or perhaps a bustling cityscape of people navigating their lives? Maybe you picture a digital landscape, where codes and algorithms govern the fabric of existence. Whatever you envisioned represents just one of the many layers of perception through which reality exists.

As we dive into the intention of an ego death, it's valuable to deconstruct reality from both external and internal perspectives, exploring its dimensions. In this way, we can uncover the profound layers that make up our experience of existence. Within the complexity lies a unique simplicity, all depending on your perspective, of course. And uncovering this simplicity amidst the complexity is your ultimate goal.

So, take a moment to gaze into the vast expanse of the seemingly small space nestled between your ears—that mysterious space that holds your flow of thoughts and collection of memories. Now, shift your focus outward and contemplate how, wherever you stand, sit, or lie, you are nestled within the boundless embrace of the universe, a tiny speck within its grandeur.

Have you ever pondered the connection between the endless horizons within your mind and the infinite reaches of the universe? Can you perceive the dual experience of our inner and outer worlds as they beautifully mirror one another?

In this exploration, we dive into the fundamental aspects of duality within reality: the internal and external, the physical and metaphysical.

We'll start at the core of it all, the physical foundation of our existence—the atom. This base layer bridges the realms of the tangible and the intangible, the seen and the unseen.

THE ATOM

At the core of our existence lies the atom, a fundamental building block that encapsulates both the external and internal realms of our reality. From the tangible elements that shape our outer world to the intricate workings of our human bodies, the atom serves as the cornerstone of our physical existence. It's awe-inspiring to realize that everything from the chair beneath you, to the food on your plate, to the air you're breathing is composed of these minuscule yet powerful entities. Yet, beyond the bounds of the material, the atom also unveils the profound beauty of our metaphysical reality, where the boundaries between the seen and unseen blur. It embodies the essence of creation, reflecting the interconnectedness of all things and opening pathways to deeper understanding and exploration of ourselves.

The atom is not immediately visible in the objects around you— the screen you're looking at or the hand you see in front of you.

But if you elevate your perspective to the microscopic realm, envisioning that every aspect of this moment is composed of countless tiny atoms, it can hopefully cultivate a deeper appreciation for your existence and the remarkable interconnectedness that makes it all possible.

Everything from humans to trees to planets exists in a fundamentally similar way, but in its own unique manner. What separates us is human thought and emotion, but recognizing our shared atomic foundation can guide us in navigating life's challenges. This interconnectedness might seem abstract at first, but consider this: once you grasp the patterns of our shared existence, the key to navigating life becomes simple. All that is left to do is understand and master your vessel—the unique character you embody.

It's during experiences like an ego-death, especially under the influence of psychedelics, that this interconnectedness can become more evident. Until then, I encourage you to elevate your perspective and contemplate this profound unity and your existence within it.

This realization isn't just a theoretical idea; quantum physics dives into some fascinating ideas about how our minds and the tiny building blocks of reality are connected. One highly intriguing experiment in physics is the double-slit experiment, which showcases how particles like electrons behave when passed through two narrow slits. These particles have a dual nature—they can behave like a wave or a particle, depending on the conditions. When no one is watching, the electron behaves like a wave, passing through both slits simultaneously. As it emerges on the other side, its wave-like nature causes it to create an interference pattern on a screen placed beyond the slits.

This pattern is similar to ripples on a pond when two stones are dropped simultaneously.

Here's where it gets mind-boggling: when scientists introduce a method to detect which slit the electron passes through (essentially watching or measuring it), the behavior changes dramatically. The electron stops behaving like a wave and starts acting like a particle, passing through just one of the slits. As a result, the interference pattern on the screen disappears, and instead, we see a pattern that resembles particles striking the screen individually—like tiny bullets hitting a target—as though the electron knows it's under observation and adjusts its behavior accordingly.

Now, this isn't just about particles behaving coyly; it hints at something much deeper. It suggests something profound about the relationship between consciousness and the physical world. It implies that our awareness, our very consciousness, has an impact on how these particles behave. This idea may seem strange, even to scientists; nonetheless, it hints at a fundamental connection between our minds and the behavior of the physical universe.

The true significance of this experiment might not strike you initially, as it seems to be about a mere shift of a particle from a wave to a dot. However, the core concept here is profound—it dives into the very essence of our existence. Consider this: the particles composing our reality are not separate from us; they are everything around us, from the air we breathe to the ground beneath our feet. What's truly astonishing is that our very attention can bring these particles to life, influencing their behavior in ways that mirror our own human experience.

When we link this mind-bending science with our journey through ego death, it's like opening a door to a whole new perspective. It shows us that our thoughts, our focus, and how we perceive things aren't just passive; they're literally active creators in shaping the world around us.

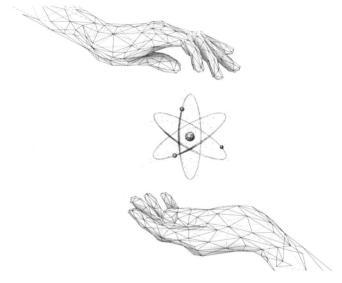

This fascinating phenomenon isn't limited to the complexities of physics; it extends seamlessly into our daily lives through the law of attraction. Have you ever heard the saying, "thoughts create things"? The double-slit experiment gives us a glimpse into this concept. Just like how particles change their behavior based on observation, our thoughts and intentions can shape our reality. Imagine atoms as tiny, responsive entities that react to our focus. When you think positively, these atoms align themselves with your desires, creating favorable outcomes in your life. This isn't just a whimsical idea; it's a profound insight into how our consciousness interacts with the world around us. This connection between our thoughts and the behavior of atoms hints at the incredible power of our minds to shape our reality.

Picture your brain as a vast network of tiny cells called neurons, constantly buzzing with electrical signals. Now, imagine each thought you have as a spark traveling through this intricate network. These sparks of thought aren't just random; they carry information and intentions. When you focus intensely on something, be it a desire, a goal, or a vision, these sparks become stronger and more focused, like beams of light cutting through the fog.

At the smallest scale, even our thoughts are made up of atoms. Quantum physics tells us that when we concentrate our thoughts and intentions on a particular outcome, we're essentially aligning these tiny particles in a way that influences the physical reality around us. You start resonating with that reality on a quantum level. The neurons in your brain fire in harmony, creating a powerful vibration that extends beyond your body and into the universe.

In this sense, manifestation isn't just wishful thinking or fantasy; it's a dynamic interplay between your conscious intentions, the firing of neurons in your brain, and the responsiveness of atoms at the quantum level. It's about tapping into the inherent creative power within you and aligning your inner world with the outer reality you wish to experience.

Understanding the power of your mind is the key to navigating through life with purpose. Being human is a complex experience, and there's much more to grasp to make our existence seem as simple as it can be.

Next, let's shift our attention into the fascinating interplay of vibration, frequency, and light—elements that emerge from the interactions of atoms and form the very foundation of our physical reality.

VIBRATIONS, FREQUENCIES & LIGHT

Exploring the realms of vibrations, frequencies, and light reveals a profound understanding that often dawns during psychedelic experiences. While not everyone may consciously recognize the nature of their experiences, there's usually an intuitive sense that arises—a deep-seated awareness of our sense of interconnectedness, a feeling that we are all one and the same. This sentiment is often echoed in psychedelic circles, where individuals express a profound sense of unity. This awareness stems from the realization that at the core of everything lie these fundamental elements: vibrations, frequencies, and light. It's as if these psychedelic journeys unveil the hidden truth that binds us all, showcasing the dance of energy that permeates every aspect of our existence.

During psychedelic experiences, the cognitive processes of our minds slow down, allowing us to perceive and grasp insights that would typically slip by our awareness. Our focus shifts to the present moment, to the sheer existence of everything around us. Unlike in our daily lives, where our attention is often occupied by various distractions, during these altered states, we become attuned to what truly matters—the essence of existence itself.

Bringing this wisdom into your psychedelic journey can profoundly transform the way you perceive and experience reality. Instead of just encountering "trippy" sensations, you'll gain a logical understanding of what you're experiencing on both a physical and mental level. This deep comprehension allows you to absorb insights in a way that changes how you see and feel about your life. Imagine not just learning about these concepts, but experiencing them in a deeply personal and tangible way. This unique and meticulous ego death journey through psychedelics will unveil the literal and delicate nature of this information, transforming it from abstract ideas into experiential truths. Your psychedelic experience then becomes more than just a fleeting moment of altered perception; it becomes a meaningful, life-changing event.

You might have noticed that in conversations about psychedelics or spirituality, terms like vibrations, frequencies, and energy come up frequently. Those who mention these concepts have experienced firsthand that these aren't abstract concepts. Ego death is an immersion into the inner workings of our being, a journey that words can't quite capture but must be felt to be truly understood.

Understanding vibrations, frequencies, and light is the next step in comprehending how our reality functions and how to navigate your existence within it. These elements play a crucial role in shaping our physical world and influence our experiences in profound ways.

Imagine the universe as a magnificent, boundless instrument, playing an eternal symphony. Think of vibrations as the underlying rhythm that permeates everything within this universal masterpiece. These vibrations, like the plucking of strings, echo through the cosmos, producing frequencies that resonate across the expanse of space.

On a grand scale, every vibration adds to the universe's harmony, like notes forming a symphony. When these frequencies align just right, they create the beautiful dance of light that shapes our reality. It's as if the universe is an orchestra, with vibrations setting the rhythm, frequencies forming the melody, and light bringing everything into focus. From the tiniest particle to the biggest star, everything plays a role in this grand cosmic performance.

Our minds function within the same magnificent framework as the universal symphony, orchestrating vibrations and frequencies that shape our reality. It's as if within us lies a miniature version of the universe's grandeur, a profound reflection of the cosmos itself. Our existence within this grand scheme is equally extraordinary, and the more we question, the more new questions arise, deepening the mystery. This is why it's my belief that psychedelics exist as a tool for transforming the incomprehensible into something experientially accessible.

During the LSD trip I previously mentioned, where I felt like a spectator within the vast realm of existence, I could hear the frequencies I was playing in my headphones and even in my thoughts echoing toward the back of my head, feeling endless, as if they could go on forever. It was like yelling into a cave or the Grand Canyon. This gave me a unique insight into the immense space within our minds and the openness required to allow such an echo. It was in this state that I realized how vibrations seem to be the physical phenomenon that makes everything else possible. Most of the energy I experienced felt almost abstract or nonexistent without the influence of these vibrations guiding the course of whatever exists.

Let's take a deeper dive into this concept with music as our tangible guide. When you strum a guitar or play a violin, you can see the strings vibrating with your naked eye. These visible vibrations are the direct manifestation of energy in motion. The movement of the strings, back and forth at rapid speeds, is a clear illustration of how vibrations work. This motion creates waves that travel through the instrument, resonating within its body. As the string vibrates, you can observe a blur or a pattern on the string, which is a physical representation of its frequency.

In a similar way, the rhythmic motion of atoms in a solid object creates its tangible form. The vibrations of these atoms are like the strummed strings of a guitar, and their rhythmic dance manifests as the solid structure and texture we can touch and see. This demonstrates the profound connection between the subtle vibrations of energy and the physical manifestation of matter. Just as each note in a symphony contributes to the whole, every atomic vibration plays a role in shaping our reality, illustrating the intricate harmony of existence.

Let's consider the example of a tree. At the core of this natural masterpiece are countless atoms vibrating at specific frequencies. These vibrations create a symphony of energy, resonating through the tree's cells and tissues. As these harmonized vibrations propagate, they interact with other factors, such as magnetic fields, gravitational forces, and molecular bonds. Imagine the vibrations within the tree's atoms moving so fast that they create the structure of the tree itself. These vibrations are not isolated; they attract and repel other energies, creating a dynamic dance that shapes the tree's form. The magnetic fields generated by these vibrations help align molecules in specific directions, while gravitational forces influence the overall stability and growth orientation of the tree. Molecular bonds act like glue, holding the atoms together in a coherent structure.

In essence, the tree emerges as a tangible manifestation of these intricate vibrational frequencies, each element contributing to the symphony of life that surrounds us. These elements, although invisible to the naked eye, are the building blocks that construct everything we see, feel, and interact with. By becoming attuned to these underlying forces, we gain a deeper understanding of how the world around us functions at its most fundamental level.

Now, let's turn our focus inward to the vibrations and frequencies within us as humans. Our entire existence is also a symphony of these subtle energies, from the rhythmic beat of our hearts to the firing of neurons in our brains. Our personal frequencies are entwined with the infinite network of frequencies in the universe.

During a psychedelic trip, these connections can become vividly apparent. You may even feel the magnetic fields that surround not only all of existence but also your own physical being, influencing your interpersonal experiences. What might seem like abstract concepts at first are actually the bedrock of reality, offering experiences that awaken a profound appreciation of existence, leading to an enlightening ego death.

Consider the emotions that course through you daily. Each emotion carries its unique energetic signature, vibrating through your body and signaling frequencies of thoughts into your mind and vice versa. Joy resonates as a vibrant hum, while sadness echoes with a softer tone. Anger may surge in sharp waves, and peace whispers in gentle ripples. These emotional energies are not mere passing moods—they are part of the cosmic orchestra playing within you, shaping your reality.

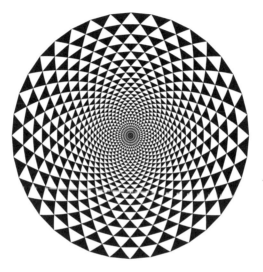

SACRED GEOMETRY

Depending on the depth and nature of your psychedelic journey, you may find yourself glimpsing these intricate patterns of frequencies that emanate from within you and manifest in your perception of reality. These patterns, often referred to as sacred geometry, are like a visual representation of the language spoken by the universe.

Sacred geometry is not just about shapes and forms. These universal patterns, seen in everything from the petals of a flower to the structure of galaxies, hint at a fundamental order and intelligence underlying the fabric of reality. They are the blueprint of our physical experience, translating the language of the universe into tangible forms. Our emotions, as powerful vibrational frequencies, contribute to this dynamic flow, creating beautifully elaborate patterns that reflect our inner states.

The experience of these geometric patterns may initially seem external, appearing on surfaces like walls or your hands. However, these frequency patterns originate from within our minds and project onto the external reality. This realization speaks volumes about the immense power within us.

This now brings us to the realm of alchemy, an ancient metaphysical science that allows us to navigate and manipulate the energy within our physical reality, offering profound insights into the nature of existence.

ALCHEMY

"As above, so below; as within, so without." This ancient principle reflects how the energies and patterns observed in the universe are mirrored in our physical reality and embodied experiences. In alchemical studies, practitioners closely examined celestial bodies, planetary movements, and metaphysical impacts, recognizing the influence of these cosmic patterns on our emotional and mental states and showcasing our interconnectedness on a grand scale.

For many, the focus of alchemy is turning base metals into gold. But this process is not just about physical transformation; it symbolizes the visible and tangible version of our goal to transmute ourselves from the lowest to the highest states. It represents the journey of turning our minds and spirits into gold—a process similar to the profound transformation experienced during an ego death. At its core, alchemy is a transformative experience that cultivates spiritual growth and understanding.

In alchemical philosophy, there's a concept known as the "prima materia," which refers to the raw material or substance from which all things are made. This prima materia isn't just physical; it encompasses the essence of everything, including our thoughts, emotions, and spiritual energy. (I like to think of this concept as the metaphysical partner of the atom, highlighting the recurring pattern of duality within our existence.) Alchemists believed that by understanding and working with the prima materia, one could initiate powerful transformations on both a physical and spiritual level.

Based on everything we've covered so far, it's evident that within our core, we are inherently connected to the fundamental elements of life. We can nurture this connection because energy exists as we do. This means that, whether we realize it or not, our lives are continually shaped and influenced by the energies of the cosmos and everything else around and within us.

Practitioners of alchemy would typically seek alignment with the natural rhythms and energies of the cosmos, striving for enhanced insight, enlightenment, and mastery over their personal reality. This transformative path involves finely tuning one's perception to the rhythmic interplay of energies, harnessing the power of sacred geometry as a direct language to intentionally manipulate vibrations and frequencies. Through this intentional practice, they seek to manifest positive outcomes and harmonize with the dynamic forces shaping the universe.

This work extends to practices such as meditation and visualization, which allow us to harness intentional energy and connect with external energies through the vibrations emitted by our minds and bodies. Our emotions constantly translate into vibrational frequencies, each creating a unique pattern that is perceived by our minds and the universe. I've found that sacred geometry helps to communicate my true intentions clearly, especially when I intend to manifest specific outcomes.

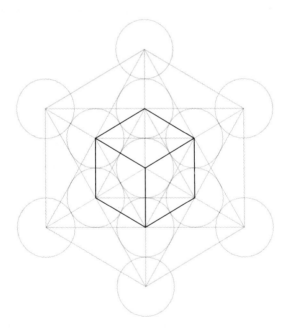

Meditation and visualization are essential tools for maintaining mental equilibrium within our rapidly processing minds. This enables us to slow down our mental processes and craft intentions with clarity, counteracting the influence of our subconscious thoughts. Our subconscious emits frequencies that the universe responds to, shaping our reality without our conscious input. Utilizing sacred geometry in meditation and visualization offers a unique advantage because it grants you the power to emit the frequencies you intend over those emitted by your subconscious.

Our minds, like sophisticated computers, store intricate memories connected to our nervous system. This delicate design makes it challenging to go against the grain of our inner thoughts and subconscious mind. When we engage with sacred geometry patterns as intentions during these practices, we gain better control over the frequencies we emit and enhance our communication with the universe. This deliberate approach enables us to harness the dynamic energies around us and steer our lives toward our true aspirations.

LIFE FORCE

Take a deep breath and connect with the pulsating energy that fuels your existence, right here and now. Feel the gentle rhythm of your heartbeat, each pulse resonating with the vitality that courses through your veins. Picture the crimson rivers of blood, carrying life's essence to every cell and organ, fueling the incredible machinery of your body. Notice the natural exchange of oxygen and carbon dioxide with each inhale and exhale.

Each breath you take is a testament to the delicate balance between life and death, as the invisible force flows in and out of your being. This life force, often referred to as "prana" in ancient traditions, is the essence that animates your existence. It's the subtle energy that connects you to the vastness of the universe. Just as the alchemists reflected on the prima materia as the raw material of creation, we can consider prana as the primal essence that bridges the gap between the physical and the spiritual realms.

Prana is perhaps one of the most undervalued treasures of our existence. It operates silently, like an invisible crutch supporting every moment of our external experience. We often overlook its significance, taking for granted its constant presence. It's easy to forget that this energy is the very essence of our vitality, the source of our true power. It's the force that allows us to move, to think, to feel, and to engage with the world around us. Yet, its duration within us remains a mystery, a delicate tether to life that should gently remind us to cherish every breath as a precious gift.

Despite our uncertainty of how long we have, we hold within us a reservoir of energy waiting to be consciously and intentionally directed. This guide toward an ego death is designed to awaken you to consciously use your life force, to channel it toward meaningful endeavors, and to infuse every action with purpose and awareness. In acknowledging the value of prana, we awaken to the beauty and fragility of our own existence, embracing each moment as a gift to be lived fully and authentically.

Our journey into the depths of life force leads us to explore the sophisticated network of energy centers, known as "the chakras," that swirl within our bodies. These chakras are like vibrant focal points where the life force pulsates with vitality and consciousness. While the physical aspect governs the tangible functions of our organs and tissues, the energetic aspect, influenced by our emotions, regulates the flow of life force through the chakras.

Let's explore the fascinating connection between our chakras and our internal functions, external experiences, and the upward flow of energy that elevates our minds and spirit.

1. Root Chakra
Location: Base of the spine
Purpose: Grounding and stability

The Root chakra anchors your energy, connecting you with the earth's energy and providing a sense of physical and emotional security. It strengthens your foundation, supporting survival instincts and grounding you in the present.

2. Sacral Chakra
Location: Just below the navel
Purpose: Creativity and emotional flow

This is the source of life's creative spark, empowering your passion, intimacy, and self-expression. The sacral chakra supports your drive to connect, create, and experience the joy that brings meaning to life.

3. Solar Plexus Chakra
Location: Upper abdomen
Purpose: Confidence and personal power

The solar plexus channels your energy into personal willpower and clarity. It's the source of your ambition, motivation, and drive to lead your life with confidence and purpose.

4. Heart Chakra

Location: Center of the chest
Purpose: Compassion and love

The heart chakra bridges the physical and spiritual aspects of your being. It channels life-force energy into love, compassion, and emotional balance, helping you to form harmonious connections with yourself and others.

5. Throat Chakra

Location: Throat
Purpose: Expression and communication

The throat chakra empowers you to speak your truth, articulate your thoughts with authentic expression and clear communication.

6. Third Eye Chakra

Location: Forehead, between the eyebrows
Purpose: Intuition

The third eye chakra channels life-force energy into intuition and insight, activating the pituitary gland to enhance perception beyond physical reality. This chakra heightens your instincts and helps you recognize deeper patterns, allowing you to trust your inner guidance and connect with life's subtler truths.

7. Crown Chakra

Location: Top of the head
Purpose: Spiritual connection and wisdom

The crown chakra is your gateway to higher consciousness, linking you to the universe and expanding your awareness beyond the self. This chakra helps you experience a sense of unity, guiding you toward enlightenment and a deeper understanding of your place in the cosmos.

The chakras form an energetic system that flows from the root chakra at the base of the spine to the crown chakra at the top of the head. This upward flow signifies our journey from physical existence to spiritual enlightenment. The chakras, interconnected and supported by each other in a harmonious dance of energy, are linked through energetic pathways called "nadis" that carry life force, or prana, throughout the body.

This energetic connection extends beyond the physical body, reaching upward to our minds and beyond. It serves as a bridge between our internal experiences and the vast intelligence of the universe, allowing us to tap into infinite wisdom, creativity, and universal consciousness.

When one or more chakras fall out of healthy alignment, disrupting this natural harmony, it severs our connection to universal intelligence. This imbalance creates a ripple effect, throwing our entire existence off balance and affecting every aspect of our reality. This means that maintaining the balance of our chakras isn't just about inner harmony; it's the key to staying attuned to the vast intelligence of the universe, ensuring a harmonious and fulfilling existence.

When our chakras are in harmonious balance, it's like having a clear and steady compass, ensuring we navigate life with clarity, purpose, and direction. The stars above us symbolize the infinite wisdom and guidance available to us when our energetic channels are open and flowing freely. However, just as clouds can obscure the stars, imbalances in our chakras can dim our connection to this cosmic intelligence, leaving us without the guidance and illumination needed to navigate the complexities of life.

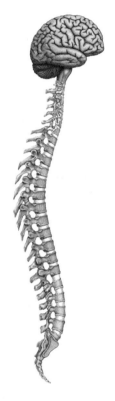

The energetic flow of our chakras is connected to our emotional energy. Negative emotions act as the main disruptors, like rocks obstructing a flowing river, causing blockages or damage within this intricate system. Envision each chakra as a radiant, swirling vortex of energy, seamlessly sending vibrations throughout your body and mind and extending into your surroundings. This flow of energy becomes an integral part of your existence, felt both internally and externally. When our emotions are harmonious and balanced, these wheels spin freely, producing an energy that fortifies our well-being.

This harmonious flow is important, because the power of our chakras lies in their ability to translate this energetic flow into action.

The mind, like a master architect, creates the blueprint of our reality—our stories, the scenes, the life experiences. Meanwhile, the body acts as the machinery that transforms the mind's intentions into tangible reality. Imagine a single idea taking shape in your mind—each thought, every intention becomes the blueprint. Your body, as the vessel for life's experiences, brings this blueprint to life, translating vision into action. By maintaining this delicate balance, we engage in a cyclical relationship where our minds and bodies work together, continuously shaping and redefining our existence, stepping into a reality created by our intentions. However, when blockages occur, disrupting this flow, our body and mind suffer, creating a disharmony that reverberates through our lived experiences.

Now let me be clear—negative emotions should not be seen as enemies of our energetic balance; rather they are essential partners to positive emotions, working together to shape our perceptions, responses, and ultimately our personal growth. It's when these negative energies remain unaddressed, untreated, and accumulate within us that they start to wield their disruptive power. Like neglected weeds in a garden, they entwine themselves with our energetic pathways, creating blockages and distortions in the natural flow of energy. This accumulated energy becomes a potent language of the body, communicating these vibrations with the mind and the universe. This cyclical relationship between mind and body continues to use these patterns to shape our reality.

When a chakra becomes disrupted or damaged, it sets off a chain reaction that can manifest as physical and emotional discomfort, and even illness. Remember, these chakras are each responsible for specific aspects of our well-being within our organs. When one of these energy centers is compromised, its corresponding physical and emotional functions may start to falter.

For instance, let's consider the heart chakra, which is closely linked with love, compassion, and emotional balance. When this vital chakra experiences disruptions or blockages, we may find ourselves grappling with emotional numbness or challenges in forming deep connections. This imbalance doesn't just affect our emotional state; it can also contribute to stress, anxiety, and depression, significantly impacting our mental and emotional well-being. Or consider an imbalance in the root chakra, which typically leads to feelings of insecurity, instability, or financial challenges, affecting our sense of safety.

On a physical level, these disruptions can also manifest as physical discomfort or illness in the related areas of the body. For instance, an imbalance in the heart chakra can lead to unexplainable pains in the chest area, affecting the heart and lungs. Similarly, an imbalance in the throat chakra, responsible for communication and self-expression, may lead to issues such as throat pain, thyroid imbalances, or speech difficulties. These disruptions in the energetic flow can also affect the surrounding chakras and their functions, creating a ripple effect throughout the entire energetic system It's like a domino effect, where one imbalance leads to another, impacting various aspects of our physical, emotional, and mental well-being.

The imbalances in our chakras continually emit our emotional frequencies, and in turn, our minds and the universe reflect or reverberate these vibrations back into our reality. This then becomes our perception of reality simply because it is what we are constantly experiencing through these vibrations. Every aspect of our reality feels the impact, from our well-being to the dynamics of our relationships and social interactions. This includes the subtle ways we perceive and engage with the world, shaping our daily experiences and the outcomes we face. Often, people traverse life's challenges without recognizing how closely their internal energy influences the external situations they draw into their lives.

When our chakras are balanced, the energy centers within us are aligned and functioning optimally. This alignment leads to a sense of clarity, inner peace, and emotional stability. By consciously maintaining this balance, we not only enhance our own well-being but also positively influence the vibrations we emit and receive, creating a more harmonious and fulfilling existence. This awareness of our energetic state and its profound influence on our reality empowers us to take an active role in shaping our lives and experiencing the world with greater depth.

EMOTIONAL INTELLIGENCE

Most of us unconsciously steer our lives through feelings and emotions, believing they're our logic, all while lacking a true understanding or connection to the depth of these emotions.

Instead, logic tends to be the primary force guiding how we live and make decisions, much like a grandmaster directing pieces on a chessboard. While relying on logic has its benefits, it often overlooks the important role emotions play in our lives. Emotions are a fundamental part of being human and significantly impact how we experience the world. We cannot escape our emotional reactions to the decisions and actions driven by logic. To fully understand the way our lives are shaped, we need to consider both logical and emotional perspectives, recognizing how they interact and influence each other.

Across generations, we've collectively struggled with neglecting our emotional well-being, and breaking this pattern demands considerable strength, given its deep roots in our societal norms. It's arguably one of the most relatable aspects of our human experience—the neglect of our emotional well-being. Only in recent times have we started openly discussing emotions, recognizing the profound impact of emotional trauma on our mental health. But I can attest that it goes even deeper than that. Acknowledging the surface aspects of our emotions is a step in the right direction, but true progress lies in unraveling the complexities and reaching the root of our emotional challenges. Our emotions are more than just words on a page; they are energies coursing through our bodies. We must unlearn much of what society and our pasts have taught us, as these experiences shape the superego and often prevent us from overriding ingrained mindsets.

Addressing and releasing the deep-seated emotions tied to our past is no small feat, but it's crucial for achieving true presence in our lives. Often, our thoughts and behaviors are not just reflections of our own experiences but are deeply rooted in generational patterns and subconscious influences. Many of us carry forward the pain and trauma from our ancestors, which shape our mindsets and actions in ways we're not always aware of. An ingrained mindset can steer our lives without us even realizing it, as we remain entangled in emotions and thoughts that aren't truly our own. To break free from these cycles and live more authentically, we must first confront these hidden influences and recognize their impact on the present moment. Our minds and bodies are tethered, with our nervous system reflecting the patterns of our past experiences. This connection can limit our ability to act in the present moment, as subconscious thoughts often influence our behavior. These automatic patterns can cause us to repeat actions or words that no longer align with our current values or needs. To truly understand ourselves and break free from these automatic responses, it's essential to actively confront and express our emotions. By doing so, we can move beyond the habitual patterns that obscure our true selves and gain a clearer, more authentic understanding of who we are.

For example, when confronting emotional trauma, it's natural to start by acknowledging what happened and how it has impacted your present life. However, simply narrating your traumas and admitting their effects isn't enough for true healing. Your inner self needs to express this emotional energy fully, in a way that may not have been possible initially. Whether it's because you couldn't fully articulate it before or because you now have a clearer understanding of yourself, it's important to readdress and release these emotions with your present perspective.

This means expressing the emotions exactly as they feel, not just what you think about them. This unfiltered expression is what we're missing. Allow yourself to fully experience and release these emotions, and you'll begin to heal in a deeper, more meaningful way. This involves diving into the complexities of our life stories, unraveling every thread to understand how each event and experience shaped us, those around us, and our perception of the world. It's about exploring the directions our emotional development took as a result of these moments, learning from the past to gain clarity and insight into our present selves. This exploration requires us to bridge the truths that are often split between our hearts and our minds. This separation creates a fragmented sense of self, with the ego holding one set of truths and the heart another. Despite how common this is, it's profoundly unhealthy, breeding distortion within our realities and making it difficult to live freely.

Our tendency to fragment our sense of self and compartmentalize our emotions often goes unnoticed, affecting both our personal lives and relationships. It's surprisingly common for us to act as if certain parts of ourselves don't exist, and this disconnection becomes so normalized that we may forget these aspects of ourselves entirely. Consequently, we become inauthentic with ourselves, making it seem normal to be inauthentic with others.

In our desire to maintain harmony and avoid discomfort, we often steer clear of deeper emotional conversations. This tendency to keep things on a surface level helps us navigate social interactions smoothly, but it can also prevent us from addressing and understanding our true feelings and those of others. We do this so naturally that we hardly notice how it normalizes emotional suppression. It's ironic because, as highly intelligent and intuitive beings, we can sense this emotional energy regardless. By ignoring our own emotions and those of our peers, we subconsciously build walls between us, adding more layers of disconnection to our reality. This widespread emotional neglect perpetuates a cycle of disconnection and inauthenticity, making true harmony and understanding difficult to achieve. We find ourselves living a distorted version of who we truly are internally—what we've become, what we could be. It's as though we're existing as a mere semblance of ourselves, not aligned with our souls, our highest selves. We wear these masks daily, a survival tactic in this cold world. At some point in our adult lives, we must recognize that our egos, which once protected us, have now become masks we've outgrown, shaping our reality into less than what we truly deserve. Ego deaths provide the chance to finally breathe outside of the suffocating falsehood that has become so normalized it's difficult to even recognize. The process of an ego death entails unraveling these layers of deception, confronting the fear that arises from admitting deep truths, and connecting with these truths. This journey is challenging because we've spent so long maintaining these facades. Ego deaths can help with embracing our emotional depth, recognizing that our emotions are not a weakness but a fundamental aspect of our realities, essential for aligning with our true selves and living authentically.

CONSCIOUSNESS, REALITY PROJECTION & PERCEPTION

Our experience of reality unfolds in a sequence: from consciousness to reality projection, and, finally, to perception. These layers or dimensions are not linear but occur simultaneously. By understanding these processes that shape our perception, we can discover how to maneuver seamlessly through the complexities of reality.

We'll start with consciousness and reality projection.

After understanding what makes up the literal fabric of our existence through energy and learning how this energy allows us to experience reality, the significance of it all lies in our ability to bridge these two forms of existence into what we experience as being human—our consciousness.

Think of your consciousness as the outlet and your capacity to project it as the plug; together, they illuminate the entirety of your human experience. The sparkling blue current of electricity flows into a socket, transferring its energy to a television. The screen flickers to life, with millions of tiny pixels lighting up in perfect synchronization, each contributing to a vivid and cohesive image. The intricate wiring and components within the television, from the speakers that produce sound to the circuits that manage color and brightness, all work together seamlessly.

Despite this straightforward system, our existence is not as obvious as it may appear to be. Recognizing our own consciousness can be challenging, primarily because we are often too busy playing our role to truly notice it. This might even seem unthinkable as you read it, but being consciously aware of our existence is difficult because we each possess different versions of ourselves that merge with varying levels of consciousness, influenced by our frequencies. These multiple selves are not something most people can easily recognize or acknowledge. Each version embodies a different perspective, emerging when a situation or emotion triggers it. It seems strange to consider that you may have multiple identities, right? But, it's true. Think of your work life, your social life, your sexual life, or your moments of solitude—all of the versions of you act and think differently, tailored to fit each situation. The compartmentalization of your psyche means there are subconscious thoughts lingering within these multiple versions of yourself, with emotions swirling through your experiences while other parts of you remain unaware.

This brings us back to the importance of perception. It is the screen of the television, the lens through which we see the world. As we go through life, we often don't consider the socket, the plug, or the sparks of electricity running through these parts. We are simply being, and as everything else operates around us, we continue to perceive life through these energies whether we realize it or not. What is in front of us is all that matters and all that we typically comprehend as it continues to shape our reality. This is why self-awareness is often elusive, it's not something you achieve by simply thinking about it.

Changing your perception requires you to change the frequency you're on. This is more than just adjusting your mood, it's about shifting the level of consciousness through which you experience life, recognizing that there are multiple levels of awareness within your reality at all moments and situations.

Imagine adjusting the dial on a radio; when aligned to the right frequency, you hear a clear and harmonious message; however, a slight misalignment results in chaotic static and distortion. Similarly, our perceptions are finely tuned to specific frequencies, meaning that only what we are tuned into exists within our field of reality. Our minds cannot perceive what doesn't exist or what we don't tune into. This is why it's crucial to elevate your level of consciousness; it allows you to see multiple and various perceptions within your reality and life. Becoming truly self-aware requires navigating these frequencies to allow your mind access to the deeper layers of your consciousness.

To begin this process, let's recognize how different frequencies resonate with and shape your consciousness. Let's take the example of being on a frequency of lust. When tuned into this vibration, your psyche can undergo a significant shift, leading to behaviors that may feel unrecognizable to your usual self. It's not just about feeling differently; this frequency can cloud your mind, obscuring other perceptions. If lust, which stems from the id's animalistic nature, combines with repressed emotions and subconscious thoughts, it can cloud your mind. This lack of self-awareness can lead to imbalanced decisions, as your logical and emotional thinking become distorted. This narrow perspective can be confusing to your other selves; you might recall instances where you were in a different frame of mind, causing you to question your actions afterward.

Now, imagine if this fog were to clear. It's as if your mind expands, allowing you to see beyond the immediate sensations of desire. This expanded awareness isn't limited to lust; it applies to all emotions. Anger, love, sadness—each emits its own frequency, altering your level of perception and consciousness. Picture your mind navigating through a dense fog, where each emotion either expands or contracts your level of awareness of yourself and reality. With an expanded level of consciousness, you can see beyond immediate emotions like a lustful mindset and also connect with the thoughts and emotions behind this mindset. This enables you to perceive the entire scenario clearly rather than just experiencing it passively, giving you greater control over your actions. At an even higher level, you can understand the language of your body and decipher what it is trying to communicate. This heightened level of consciousness allows you to direct your body's responses, rather than being driven by them. By allowing yourself to see beyond the immediate emotions, your consciousness expands, enabling you to consider more aspects of yourself and your reality.

At first glance, this might seem uncomplicated. However, it's important to understand that shifting your level of consciousness isn't a purely mental experience—it ripples through your entire physical reality, a reality built on magnetic energy that responds to your internal state.

THE ROLE OF EMOTIONS IN THE SPECTRUM OF CONSCIOUSNESS

Now, I want you to remember when you were younger, newly captivated by the allure of two magnets and the mysterious space of energy between them. Recall the sensation of that energy taking an invisible shape, the push and pull as you maneuvered the magnets, aligning or repelling them with force. We are experiencing the exact same thing in our daily lives, just on an incredibly large scale. Imagine substantial spaces of energy formed around you, working in the exact same way, influencing and shaping our experiences every single day.

Our bodies have three layers of magnetic fields, like rings of energy surrounding us, each with significant spaces between them. Each barrier leads to the next tier of magnetic energy, influencing and shaping our levels of consciousness. The closest tier to our bodies aligns with our emotional consciousness. This tier forms the foundation where our reality is shaped by our feelings, creating deeply personal and intimate perceptions of the world. (The next tier, connected to the third eye, is where your intuitive and divine self communicates between the highest and lowest versions of you. Finally, the outermost tier is the soul level, representing your infinite, energetic essence—the purest form of your being, where you exist as divine energy itself.)

You may recognize this energy within yourself during moments of strong emotions. For example, during a fragile and vulnerable moment, you may unexpectedly feel yourself welling up to cry. A heavy sensation surrounds your head, traveling down to your throat, making it difficult to speak clearly. This deep emotion creates a friction that feels like heat radiating around your ears and then enveloping your entire body. This is just one example of the powerful and clearly physical impact of our emotional frequency. In moments of vulnerability, when we allow our mind to briefly embrace thoughts that evoke strong emotions, we come face to face with the raw intensity of those emotions. Whether we acknowledge them or not, our emotions are always present—but it's in the direct confrontation of these feelings that we experience the undeniably powerful, tangible reality they bring, dramatically different from the muted reality where they remain hidden.

The magnetic force of energy encircling us as the emotions take over allows our minds to momentarily enter this expansive energy realm and witness its power.

WHAT IS EMOTIONAL CONSCIOUSNESS?

Naturally, when reflecting on our emotions, we tend to focus on intense or dramatic feelings. However, we may overlook the quieter ways emotions subtly guide our thought processes. When we are tuned in to emotional consciousness, we often find ourselves projecting.

Projection means seeing a reflection of your personal experiences, views, and feelings in situations outside of yourself. This can happen in many different ways. The problem with projection is that it prevents you from seeing the truth of what's in front of you. Instead, it's like you're reliving a memory or reacting from feelings in situations that aren't exactly related, but to you, they feel that way.

Emotional consciousness can also hold us back from embracing new ideas or trying new things. Your thoughts tend to lead you toward what feels natural, safe, or predictably comfortable, keeping you confined within familiar boundaries. Remember, our reality shifts to what we focus our energy on, but what we focus on isn't always within our conscious thoughts. Our thoughts are incredibly fast, and it can be hard to catch them all. Often, we don't recognize that a thought came from our emotional consciousness because that emotion isn't within our full awareness.

For example, there is a disabled man with cerebral palsy who decided to try standup comedy. He evidently enjoys making fun of himself and while doing his set he encouraged fellow comedians to unleash their humor while he joined in, laughing along. But in the audience, there was a man who got triggered. This particular man clearly wasn't fully present at this moment. Instead, he began to project something deep within himself, leaving the collective reality of the comedy room and viewing this situation with his emotional consciousness. Now there can be a number of reasons something sparked within him that made him, view this scene in a way that caused him to get upset and offended. Perhaps he recalls a memory of a time when someone made fun of him or someone he loved, in a similar way. Or it can be even deeper, stemming from the depths of the subconscious mind. For instance, he might have felt triggered because he found the jokes humorous but believed it was inappropriate to laugh. Instead of embracing the humor, he got upset at the idea of it all, driven by a subconscious desire to be seen as a good person—based on yet another subconscious thought driven by a suppressed emotion. This shows how our subconscious thoughts can creep into our thinking at any moment, shaping our reactions and perceptions without us even realizing it. In his mind, this experience was offensive and upsetting, compelling him to interrupt the show and express his disapproval. He even offered apologetic compassion to the disabled comedian, praising him for his bravery. On the surface, this might seem like the behavior of a considerate person, but if we view the scenario from the comedian's perspective, a different story unfolds. The comedian didn't want to be singled out and treated sensitively because of his condition—perhaps he had experienced enough of that throughout his life. In this moment, he wanted to have fun, let loose, and be part of something beyond his disability. This was evident in his demeanor and sense of humor; however, the audience member's feelings distorted the reality of the situation. He couldn't be present and recognize the experience unfolding before him; he could only perceive what he felt. This example shows how our emotional consciousness can hijack our perception, steering us away from the reality in front of us and into our own deeply personal experiences and reactions.

Another common and relatable experience of projection is seen in the parent-child relationship, where the parent's past experiences, emotions, and subconscious thoughts significantly influence their behavior and interactions with their child. These influences can shape the parent's expectations, the way they treat their child, and even their perception of the child's identity. Sometimes, parents may unknowingly impose their own life experiences onto their children, expecting them to follow certain paths or behave in specific ways based on the parent's own upbringing. This can lead to a limited understanding of the child's individuality and unique personality, as the parent may only see life through their own lens of experiences and emotions.

This pattern of projection is quite common. Naturally, we interpret the world around us based on our own thoughts, feelings, and beliefs. However, when this perception is intertwined with suppressed emotions and unaddressed subconscious thoughts, it can lead us deeper into the realms of emotional consciousness. In this state, we may act and make decisions based on underlying emotions and past experiences, often without realizing the extent to which they influence our interactions with others.

Think of it this way: your body is not just a physical form; it's the very conduit that connects you to the world. Now, within and around this physical vessel, there exists a subtle yet powerful magnetic energy. This energy isn't something you can touch or see, but it's there, intimately intertwined with your being.

This magnetic force is like a bridge between your body and your thoughts. It's what allows you to feel the warmth of a hug, the rush of excitement, or the pang of sadness. When you experience these emotions, it's not your thoughts doing the feeling—it's your body. Your body is the one registering these sensations and sending signals to your mind. Now, here's where it gets interesting. This magnetic energy doesn't just stop at the body; it extends into your mind, influencing the flow of your thoughts. Our emotions, sensations, and thoughts are all intertwined within this magnetic field, creating a continuous loop where how we feel informs how we think, and vice versa. Imagine it as a stream of consciousness, where your emotions act as the currents guiding the direction of your thoughts. When you're feeling joyful, your thoughts may flow effortlessly, focusing on positive aspects of life. Conversely, during moments of stress or sadness, this magnetic energy can create turbulence in your thought stream, leading to anxious or negative thoughts. The key here is awareness As long as we allow ourselves to be immersed in this field, our minds remain attuned to this blend of physical and emotional consciousness.

THIRD-EYE CONSCIOUSNESS

There are approximately 6 meters of emotional energy surrounding your body. This is more significant than it may sound. Magnetic fields operate just like the smaller magnets I mentioned earlier. So, when you consider that small force field of energy between two tiny magnets, can you imagine the immense force and power that surrounds your human body?

This force field forms a powerful barrier to the next tier of consciousness—your logical, or "third-eye" consciousness. The effort required to break through to this higher level of consciousness demands immense emotional strength and mental power, as it means overcoming the physical emotional frequency that governs your thoughts to obtain genuine clarity needed to observe your life through your third eye. Transcending your current state of awareness via ego death isn't just about understanding yourself; it's about realizing the profound strength within you and using it to transcend and expand your consciousness.

Navigating through the intense energy of your emotional world is like braving a tumultuous sea. It feels as though you're pushing through powerful waves, each one larger than the last, overwhelming in their strength. What makes this energy even more formidable is not just its power but also the cunning strength of your ego. Going against this force feels like entering a danger zone, as the ego fiercely guards its version of reality. It detests the idea of any vulnerability, fearing exposure that could lead to discomfort or pain. Yet, embracing this challenge is the pathway to a new level of consciousness, expanding your awareness beyond the confines of structured mindsets. It opens the door to seeing life in a completely new and liberating way, free from the constraints of ego-driven perceptions.

Once you free yourself by gaining control over your emotional energy, rather than letting it control you, you can maneuver your focus and shift your level of perception and consciousness with ease and grace.

CHANGING PERCEPTION THROUGH NEW PERSPECTIVES

Shifting your perception is quite different from shifting your level of consciousness. Changing your perception is about altering your perspective, which can be relatively straightforward by adjusting your point of view. However, shifting your level of consciousness goes deeper, leading to a profound transformation in how you perceive, interpret, and engage with the world. It's not just about seeing things differently; it's about experiencing a new level of understanding and connection to reality.

Using psychedelics offers a direct and profound route to altered and elevated states of consciousness. However, until then, changing your perspective remains a valuable and accessible method to maneuver our perception of reality. While shifting your level of consciousness requires significant effort, even just changing your perspective can lead to heightened awareness.

Perception and perspective are like two sides of the same coin: perception is the lens through which we see reality, and perspective is the angle from which we view it. By changing our perspective, we can effectively shift our perception of life.

So, let's explore the art of shifting perspectives by imagining that the television that represents your mind has a unique dial with three options for perception: first, second, and third person. As you turn the dial to the first-person perspective, the screen fills with vivid images of your own experiences and emotions. From this angle, everything you interpret is filtered through your emotions and beliefs about yourself, others, and the world around you. Your perception becomes a projection of your inner reality. This means that the experiences you encounter often reflect the same truths you hold within yourself. Your feelings and thoughts cloud your judgment, leading you to assume that the same frame of mind applies to everything around you.

Next, you flip the switch to the second-person perspective. As the screen transitions, you may still feel emotions deeply, but these emotions no longer define your entire perception of reality. Instead, you gain a clearer understanding of your role within the roles of others. You pay closer attention to your actions and behaviors, noticing how they impact those around you. This heightened awareness also reveals how external influences shape your behavior, feelings, and ultimately, your reality. This second-person perspective allows for clearer self-reflection .

Finally, you flip the switch to the third-person perspective. The screen widens to reveal a panoramic view of your life, detached yet comprehensive. From this vantage point, you gain a deeper understanding of the interconnectedness of events, the patterns that emerge, and the broader context of your experiences. This expanded perspective allows you to practice more control over your life, as you grasp the full scope of your reality. You see the roles you play in various situations with clarity, making your actions and decisions more intentional and impactful. With this heightened insight, you can navigate challenges more effectively, leverage opportunities to your advantage, and create a life that aligns with your values and aspirations.

The farther you can see outside of your own emotions, the greater your understanding and adaptability, leading to profound growth. Consider that shifting your perspective is the pathway toward elevating your consciousness. Our perspectives shift and change with the events and situations in our lives, influenced by our varying values and experiences. In contrast, consciousness reflects a way of life—it's your constant mindset and awareness.

Living without the intrusive influence of the ego marks a significant shift in consciousness. Once you connect with your highest self, the journey through life becomes progressively smoother. It's a state where you're simultaneously aware of yourself—your emotions, reactions, and thoughts—alongside a keen perception of your surroundings and others' behaviors. This heightened awareness allows you to make decisions that genuinely benefit your life, free from the constraints of ego-driven impulses and habitual patterns. This expanded consciousness grants you the wisdom to recognize your interconnectedness with the vastness of the universe. You begin to see yourself not as separate from the world but as an integral part of it, guided by universal truths rather than ego-driven desires. This shift allows you to navigate life with clarity and purpose, each decision becoming a manifestation of this elevated consciousness, shaping a reality aligned with your highest ideals and deepest truths.

THE 1-3-2 METHOD

While higher consciousness grants us greater insight into our emotions, reactions, and thoughts, it's important to recognize the fine line between having awareness and having control of intense emotions. Emotions serve as our guiding compass in life, and attaining higher consciousness does not mean disconnecting from them. In the process of shifting our consciousness, we learn to harness the power of emotions without letting them overwhelm or control us. The journey involves deepening our understanding of ourselves—a process that unfolds gradually, with practice, over time. This transformation is not instantaneous, especially considering the immense power of our subconscious mind. This aspect cannot be overstated; to navigate this journey, honing your ability to communicate with your body and interpret its signals is essential. Equally important is cultivating a balanced mindset. I stumbled upon a valuable insight during an introspective journey with LSD—a framework I call the 1-3-2 method. This method has been instrumental in navigating the complexities of our conscious dimensions.

The 1-3-2 method involves identifying each of the three levels of yourself as distinct personas, allowing you to become much more aware of your behaviors and frequency.

Throughout my psychedelic journeys, I found myself becoming extremely clear with my inner selves. It was a natural realization that my everyday self—the one living life based on subconscious patterns, inner wounds, and personality tendencies—was the lowest version of me, which I labeled as Level 2.

The higher version of myself that I experienced on LSD wasn't a stranger. It wasn't that LSD made me act or think differently; I simply saw my life, myself, and my actions with profound clarity. This version literally felt elevated, and the number 3 strongly resonated with this level of mind. The number 3 kept appearing in my mind, resonating with an undeniable truth that I couldn't ignore. It felt as though this knowledge had always been within me, just waiting to be rediscovered.

Then, during a completely different experience, I found myself repeatedly saying the number 1 as I connected deeply with my highest self. I remember talking, and wisdom I had never spoken of before was just pouring out of my mouth. My mind was so focused that every few minutes, I would hear myself speaking in another frequency, noticing that I kept repeating the number 1. Then, something snapped, making me realize that this number 1 was crucial in understanding the version of myself I was experiencing at that very moment. I felt a profound simplicity, especially when compared to my lowest self, which viewed life so complicatedly. I found that as I comprehended this insight, it naturally and seamlessly became ingrained within me.

By visualizing these different levels, you can better understand your behaviors and align more closely with your highest self. The 1-3-2 method helps you navigate your thoughts and emotions, bringing you closer to a state of heightened awareness. You might assume that my lowest self would be labeled as "1," but these identifications aren't based on a structured order. Instead, they're labeled by their dimension of self-reflection.

Let me explain: 2 represents your physical self, where everything you experience is through your own perspective—your character. An easy way to remember this is that you see life with your two eyes, and your mind can only perceive what the eyes tell it to. The connection between your eyes, brain, and heart forms a delicate relationship that typically experiences life on a two-dimensional level. To put it simply, these two dimensions are yourself and the reality before you.

Then we have the Level 3 persona. Think of this version of yourself as your "third-eye self." Your third-eye has its own perception of yourself, life, and the world, which can feel as though these perceptions are separate from your lower self. In reality, it's an expanded awareness that is intimately connected with the universe. The third eye, scientifically known as the pineal gland, plays a crucial role in this deeper insight into life and reality.

> Located in the center of the brain, the pineal gland is a gateway to higher consciousness and is known as a point of intuition, spiritual insight, and connection to the universe. When activated, it transcends ordinary perception, allowing you to experience a profound sense of unity with the universe and access deeper layers of consciousness.

Finally, we come to Level 1, which I experienced with remarkable clarity while sitting in the middle of a forest, simply enjoying the moment and unraveling the complexities of our existence with ease. This level resonates as the highest self because it is a combination of both your second self and your third self. It is metaphysical math, where you incorporate all dimensions of thinking and being all that you are capable of— united into one full perspective of your reality. This version of you is an embodiment of a piece of the cosmos living its experience through you. It's an integrative state where the physical, mental, and spiritual aspects converge, creating a sense of wholeness and unity with the universe.

The order of our consciousness levels, starting from the physical body, is naturally in the sequence of 2, 3, 1. But I call it the 1-3-2 method because this is the alignment that allows me to view life from the highest level of perception. Whenever I make decisions or reflect on my life, I begin with the perspective of my highest self—the "1"—because this version of me is directly connected to the universe. It sees the bigger picture and always has my best interest at heart. Then, the "3"—my third eye self—acts as the mediator, filtering how my emotional self will understand and process what's coming. Finally, the "2," my emotional self, responds and reacts to the filtered information in a way that resonates with my feelings and physical experiences. I've even given each of these versions a name to better connect with and understand them, reinforcing how each one plays a role in how I navigate life and stay aware of my behavior.

AS ABOVE, SO BELOW, AS WITHIN, SO WITHOUT

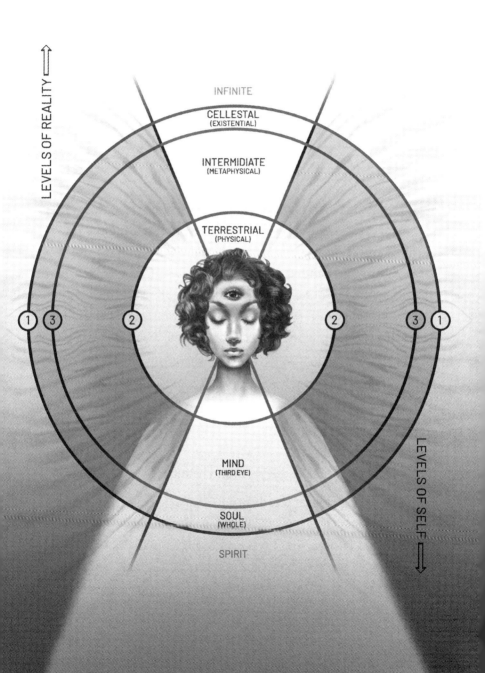

LEVELS OF REALITY

LEVELS OF SELF

INFINITE

CELLESTAL
(EXISTENTIAL)

INTERMIDIATE
(METAPHYSICAL)

TERRESTRIAL
(PHYSICAL)

1 3 2 2 3 1

MIND
(THIRD EYE)

SOUL
(WHOLE)

SPIRIT

CHAPTER 4

✴ ☽ ✴

THE JOURNEY
OF THE SOUL

This voyage has taken you from the vastness of the cosmos to the intimate dance of molecules within you, revealing the profound connection between the external energies and the life force within. As each piece of wisdom about our reality weaves its way from the outer realms, it flows seamlessly into your being, merging with your essence. From there, it gracefully cycles back out into the world, forming a harmonious link between your inner experience and the external reality.

Consider the profound capability your mind holds to organize and comprehend the entirety of our existence through thought alone. This is where you can witness, in this very moment, the essence of who you truly are. Open your heart to the wisdom of your journey and feel the profound beauty of your existence.

At the heart of all existence, deep within us, lies the essence and life force that sustains us. The profound depth of your inner thoughts, your capacity to feel and to be, is made possible by the soul that was uniquely paired with the life and body you now inhabit. This is the most important part of your existence.

Everything else we have discussed pertains to the functionality and operations of our existence within reality, but your soul is the key to it all. It is the soul that gives life its depth and meaning, that connects you to the grand design of existence. It is your soul, your innermost essence, that truly defines you and guides you through the intricate dance of life.

As you step closer to Part 2 of this guide, may your heart be open and your soul receptive to the profound transformation ahead. Every piece of wisdom you've absorbed has woven itself into the fabric of your being, preparing you for the depths of introspection that await during your psychedelic exploration.

In this sacred space of self-discovery, allow your mind to soften its grip, granting your soul the freedom to guide your experience. It can be a challenging shift, as the mind has long held sway over your thoughts and actions. Yet, surrendering to the flow of your true essence is the key to unlocking the door to a life renewed after ego death.

As you traverse the realms of your inner world, may you be enveloped in a sense of openness and connection to your soul's wisdom. Acknowledge the truths of your reality, cherish the miracle of your existence, and let your innermost thoughts merge harmoniously with the whispers of your soul. The delicate balance between mind and soul serves as a gateway to profound self-awareness and a deeper comprehension of life's purpose and beauty.

Before you embark on your journey, remember this: the complexities of existence coexist harmoniously with the simplicities of life. Consider this chapter as a touchstone—a reminder of life's fundamental truths and simplicities. Whenever you feel overwhelmed by the chaos of the external world, return to the words you'll find here. Let them serve as your anchor, guiding you back to the essence of your being, offering clarity and perspective as you navigate your transformative journey.

It's important that you establish what's important to your soul, what resonates deeply with your heart, and to understand yourself on a deeper level entirely. Life often splits us between who we have to be—shaped by our jobs, families, and societal expectations—and who we intrinsically are. This journey is an opportunity to grasp the clarity of who you truly are and who you've become. Embrace this moment to reconnect with your authentic self, to recognize the divergence between your external roles and your inner essence. By doing so, your everyday self will align more closely with your true nature, paving the way for a more profound and meaningful existence.

YOUR LIFE'S MASTERPIECE

Remember, in life you are not merely a participant but the esteemed director and the main character. Despite the moments that may seem beyond your control, remember the power you possess to shape the narrative. Your life is the most significant narrative you will ever create. Each day presents a canvas for your creativity, a stage for your choices.

Pause and think to yourself: if you were to watch the movie of your life, would it be one you'd eagerly watch? What moments, what virtues, what actions would evoke pride, joy, and contentment? As you reflect on your story, deeply consider all the roles you play. Are you proud of each role and how you fulfill it? What has been shaping your narrative so far? Is this the storyline you wish to continue, or is it time to take control and craft a movie that brings you joy in every scene of living? Reflect on whether you are embodying the best version of yourself in each role and make intentional choices that align with the story your soul would truly want to tell.

This is not a mere exercise; this is a compass guiding you toward a life lived with intentionality. The heart of this message lies in acknowledging that this journey is yours to navigate. While external forces may influence the plot, your responses, decisions, and perspectives shape the reality of your life. It can be tricky to distinguish between what's most important to your character versus what's essential for your soul. Keep your mind and heart in balance, and always listen to the nudges from your heart. It's not about creating a flawless script but about infusing each scene with authenticity, resilience, and compassion. Embrace the imperfections, because they are the brushstrokes that give depth to your story. As you reflect on your life's narrative, remember that the most profound satisfaction comes from living authentically, loving fiercely, and embracing the beauty of your unique journey.

THE ART OF HAPPINESS

What is happiness if not the soul's contentment? Happiness is more than just a passing feeling; it's a state of being that you cultivate through intentional actions and choices. The journey of the soul challenges the allure of comfort and convenience. Instead, the soul seeks to use the heart in ways that make it flutter with joy, grow warm with excitement, and express love uniquely.

True happiness comes from creating moments that resonate deeply with who you are. It involves embracing experiences that fill you with genuine joy and fulfillment. Happiness can be found in both simple and grand moments, and it's up to you to create these opportunities. Remember, you cannot wait for happiness to come to you, nor can you rely on others to make you happy. You must take control of your happiness, starting with gratitude for your life. Acknowledge the blessing of being alive and let this gratitude lead you toward what is possible. Because you have the privilege of time within your body, use it to experience things that bring you joy. This is the essence of true happiness: actively seeking and creating experiences that make your soul come alive.

FREE WILL

Free will is a delicate concept, best understood in moments of profound introspection, especially during a psychedelic experience. Imagine free will as being the space beyond the door unlocked by an ego death. Picture this door as a threshold to a world unbounded by the constraints of the mind. On one side of this door lies a labyrinth of walls and corridors that confine thoughts, beliefs, and perceptions within a finite framework of understanding. It's a space where the echoes of conditioning and societal norms reverberate, whispering limitations and boundaries. But step through that door, and you step into the vastness of free will.

In the transformative moment of an ego death, you journey full circle, 360 degrees, back to the essence of your being—a pure soul, unencumbered by constructs, simply experiencing life. The person you have become is a culmination of your experiences, yet at your core, your soul remains pure and free, devoid of attachments, and thus capable of creating infinite possibilities.

Free will seems daunting to a version of you that clings to answers, reasons, and excuses that justify your actions—a reflex of the ego striving to know and validate your existence in familiar ways. However, after an ego death, the realization dawns that your mind shapes the reality you experience, placing the responsibility squarely on your shoulders. From that moment forward, the responsibility is yours to wield the vast potential of your mind. It's no longer about simply existing within the confines of conditioned responses and societal norms; it's about actively creating your reality, embracing the unknown, and stepping into the limitless potential of your soul.

Your mind is the most potent tool at your disposal, and it's entirely within your control. However, every thought, every belief, every boundary within your mind holds sway over your consciousness; even the smallest thought imposes limitations within your mind, wielding more control than you realize. After a lifetime of thinking a certain way and holding onto beliefs, it can be challenging to let go. Yet, the price of clinging to old patterns is heavy—it continuously constrains the freedom your mind is designed for. Truly consider how much of all that you know controls your thoughts and dictates your way of life. Everything you've learned up until this moment has likely been beneficial, shaping your journey and guiding you through the complexities of your story. Your old mindset served a purpose, leading you to where you were destined to be. But continuing with the same mindset, knowing deep within that you have a higher purpose and limitless potential, would render this path aimless. Now, you stand at the threshold of a new understanding, where you can wield the power of your mind to experience life as you were designed to—freely and abundantly.

Facing these truths can still be difficult to understand without experiencing the power of your mind on your own. It's understandable that holding such power within you might seem unbelievable or intimidating. You may find yourself thinking, "How does this align with my existing beliefs? What if I lose my grip on reality?" It's natural to have doubts and questions when faced with the idea of letting go of everything that seems to define your entire existence. However, it's crucial to remember that your grip on reality will never be outside of your control. Everything within your conscious awareness is under your command, and as you continue on this journey, you will learn more about how to wield this control.

Tell yourself now that you are challenging these fears by continually exploring the vastness of your mind. This exploration is nothing to fear; any hesitation arises from confronting the unknown. Fear of the unknown is natural, but rather than seeing the unknown as intimidating, envision it as a blank canvas awaiting your creativity. Remember, exploring your mind is your birthright. It's your own sanctuary, a gift to experience your life fully. No one and nothing should have power over it but you. Embrace this journey, release all fear, and take control with courage and curiosity.

This introspection will guide you to understand the divinity within your existence, allowing you to touch greatness with thought alone. As you move forward in this guide, you will find that your ability to navigate and shape your reality grows stronger, empowering you to embrace the profound depths of your consciousness.

The philosophical question, "If a tree falls in a forest and no one is around to hear it, does it make a sound?" is not meant to spark debate but to awaken the depths of your consciousness. It's a powerful reminder that your mind is a microcosm of the universe, and you are uniquely experiencing the vastness of existence through your own lens. Every aspect of your reality— the place you live, the people you surround yourself with, the information you consume—exists because you perceive it. Consciousness means being aware, and it's this awareness that gives life to sounds, touches, sights, and all other senses. Without your awareness, these experiences simply don't exist. When something enters your consciousness, it becomes alive, but only as alive as you allow it to be. So, does the falling tree exist if it's not witnessed, heard, or felt? No, it does not. Your reality is shaped entirely by what you allow into it.

BALANCE WITHIN DUALITY

As we've already covered, life is characterized by a pervasive pattern of duality. Everywhere we look, we encounter pairs—up and down, left and right, in and out, light and dark, good and bad. This duality is part of the divine balance of existence.

Being human can feel like both a blessing and a burden; it's in the gray areas of life, where opposites meet, that we find the true richness of our experiences. Here, we are able to enjoy what life has to offer rather than just going through the motions. Navigating this gray area is both an art and a science. We can consider the artistic aspect of life through the heart, embracing creativity, intuition, and emotion, while the scientific aspect filters through the mind, applying logic, reason, and analysis. Balancing these dimensions allows us to fully experience the depth and richness of our existence. This explains why relying solely on our personalities to navigate life isn't as efficient. Our personalities act as specific lenses—whether you're an introvert or extrovert, whether you lean more on logic or intuition—limiting us to a narrow perspective. True balance means mindfully choosing to see the entirety of our experiences as we live them, beyond the confines of our habitual tendencies.

Living in balance can feel like a constant process of fine-tuning ourselves. Our emotions and thoughts are in constant flux, shaped not only by our internal dynamics but also by external energies. Consider how you may think and feel differently during the night compared to the day, a reflection of the energies of the sun and moon influencing us. Even the days of the week are aligned with certain planets, each exerting its unique impact on us. It's important to continuously be mindful and fine-tune our thought processes and emotions because this mirrors how the universe operates. The universe is always in flux, with things shifting and changing daily based on various cosmic forces. In recognizing this pattern of duality, we can understand that we operate in a similar fashion—a microcosm of the macrocosm. By acknowledging and embracing this relationship with the universe, we can navigate life's ebbs and flows with greater awareness and harmony.

Maintaining this equilibrium allows us to navigate life without losing sight of the bigger picture of our reality and story. When we become too imbalanced on the emotional side, we risk getting immersed in our character or experiences, missing out on the details that shape our story and the opportunities to intentionally impact it. Conversely, if we lean too heavily on the logical side, we may overlook the details of our lives that shape our story and miss opportunities to create beauty and purpose. Finding this delicate equilibrium allows us to live life without becoming too detached from the present or losing the richness and depth of our experiences.

In this delicate balance, we come to see that our souls possess two centers of wisdom: the heart and the brain. They are like two different individuals coexisting within your single body. Trusting every aspect of who you are is crucial. Allowing these parts to communicate with each other is the first step toward creating harmony within your life. By recognizing and nurturing this internal conversation, you foster a deeper connection to your true self, enabling you to navigate life with confidence and clarity.

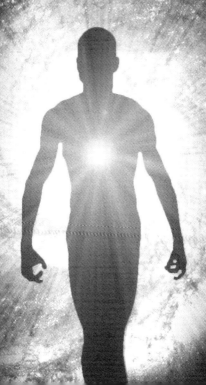

PART 2

EGO DEATH—CHARTING THE COURSE TO SELF-REBIRTH

※ ☽ ※

CHAPTER 5

ALIGNING PSYCHEDELIC CHOICES WITH GOALS

Welcome to the journey ahead, one that promises liberation and rejuvenation at every turn. Before we dive into the depths of ego death, it's crucial to understand where you currently stand on this transformative path. Just as life and being human are multifaceted, so too is the process of ego death. It's not a one-size-fits-all experience; rather, it unfolds in layers, each revealing deeper aspects of yourself. Knowing where you need support and guidance is key to safely and effectively unraveling your ego. Think of it as exploring different trails to reach hidden treasures within yourself. Unraveling these layers requires careful navigation and introspection, recognizing the unique challenges and opportunities that each layer presents. Our journey together is about finding the right paths to unlock your innermost truths and pave the way for a profound transformation.

Before we begin, I want to highlight a crucial point as both your guide and fellow psychonaut—I firmly believe there's a profound distinction between drugs and psychedelics. Just as there's a spectrum to describe our human minds, the term "drug" feels like an umbrella term that doesn't quite capture the transformative experiences psychedelics bring, unlike other substances that can deplete you.

Now, I'm not one to endorse a lifestyle where substance abuse is the norm. If you happen to mix substances, I suggest considering a pause for this guide. This way, your mind and body won't be overstimulated, allowing you to extract the utmost from your experiences. By the end of this journey, you'll understand yourself in a way that might make you question the need for mixing substances in the first place and gain deeper insights into why you feel the urge to do so. For those who've never tried any substances or aren't very familiar with this world of mind alterations, you've come to the right guide. I'm all about safe, clean, and effective tripping, and my goal is to guide you to where you're destined to be—exploring the rhythm of your psyche more than the psychedelics themselves.

Moving on, my explorations have involved three forms of psychedelics: psilocybin, LSD, and ayahuasca. While I'm eager to explore DMT, a psychedelic that's known as a gateway to other dimensions, and San Pedro, a cactus known for its heart-opening effects, they remain uncharted territory for me. As a result, my focus will revolve around the three companions that have significantly enriched my journeys toward enlightenment.

Much like choosing the mode of transportation for a physical trip, opting for a specific psychedelic substance defines the nature of your exploratory experience. Like a traveler exploring the unknown, these psychedelic journeys are packed with experiences that can enrich your understanding of life and yourself. Just as returning from travels often brings change, your voyage into the realms of the mind, body, and spirit is likely to leave an indelible mark on your life.

I've assigned each psychedelic a personality that dictates how it effectively elevates you and in which aspect of yourself you'll experience a lift. The type of psychedelic you choose can significantly influence your perception. Your mind and energy are malleable, and psychedelics can enhance one aspect more than another. So, let me break down how these different worlds are experienced based on the type of psychedelic.

PSYCHEDELIC "PERSONALITIES"

PSILOCYBIN, OR "MAGIC MUSHROOMS"

Imagine psilocybin as the intuitive and nurturing mother. She's all about guiding you vibrationally, showing you the way to a deeper understanding of your existence. Picture her as a journey into the soul, where emotions are heightened and awareness is finely tuned to the physical self and the surrounding reality. Mama psilocybin also reveals the heart-centered connections between yourself and the energies surrounding you. She doesn't just show you what's physically present; she delicately highlights the intuitive aspects often overlooked in your daily life. This emotionally driven experience becomes a bridge, connecting you to inner truths and the emotions attached to these truths. She is your guide to your reality, unveiling the essence of your existence through your own vibrations.

LSD, OR "ACID"

LSD is like the wise and insightful father, offering a profound glimpse behind the veil of reality. Father LSD is a blunt and straightforward guide to navigating the inner workings behind the scenes of life—he is the middleman between your highest and lower selves. Driven by logic, Father LSD uncovers the intricate blueprint of existence. Under his influence, the vast power of your mind comes to light, revealing layers of consciousness that may have been hidden before. He emanates raw power, guiding you to recognize and wield the inherent strength you delicately hold. It's a journey where the boundaries of reality stretch and the complexity of your existence becomes clearer. This journey can illuminate the pathways to navigate the physical world more effortlessly and align your multidimensional selves with a unified mindset.

AYAHUASCA, OR "VINE OF THE SOUL"

Enter ayahuasca, the mystical grandmother of the psychedelic family, a beacon of profound spiritual experiences. This potent brew, often recognized as a deeply spiritual experience to partake in, takes on a nurturing role, personifying the wisdom of an ancient grandmother guiding her kin. Grandmother Ayahuasca is a healer who tenderly rubs your back as you vulnerably surrender to her divinely orchestrated process. In the sacred space she creates, ayahuasca is more than a mere purge; she's a divine remedy, gently coaxing you to surrender and release what no longer serves your soul. As you vulnerably lean into her, ayahuasca's presence becomes a comforting embrace, offering solace as the cleansing unfolds. The purge becomes a cathartic release of emotional burdens and stale or toxic energies. As ayahuasca cradles your wounded self, you find solace in the cleansing ritual, symbolizing not just a physical release but a spiritual rebirth. In her grandmotherly wisdom, ayahuasca becomes the compassionate guide, soothing your inner self from the inside out. This is not a mere psychedelic encounter; it's a conversation with the divine.

While each of these options holds its own merits, their usefulness depends on your current stage of personal development and your specific intentions. Whether you choose one or plan to explore all three, it's crucial to consider the structure of your journey. If you're a seasoned psychonaut you may be thinking, "There is no need for so much planning and detail for such a freeing experience." A younger, less wise version of myself would agree with that; however, I've learned that preparing the journey for your physical self (or two-dimensional self) is extremely important when looking for effective transformation from these experiences. Yes, these psychedelic experiences can bring you profound liberation, but they can also be limited to a temporary liberation if you don't understand how to embody that experience. Exploring your mind is a delicate art, and embracing the genius within you lies in seamlessly integrating these experiences into your daily life. Everyone has a unique story they're playing out, so it may be necessary to see new angles of your life or experience through a deepened conscious perspective, or high consciousness, that enriches your self-perception. Beyond the initial feeling of freedom, there's a deeper journey that can benefit your life.

Whether your choices are guided by intuition or sparked by curiosity about certain psychedelics, aligning your starting point with confidence requires a deep understanding of your present mental and emotional states. Delving into the intricacies of your mind, heart, and spirit will not only bring clarity to your current state but also guide you toward the psychedelic experience that resonates most with your personal growth objectives.

The following questions are your compass, offering general insights to categorize where you stand in your unique journey. These will pave the way to determine the perfect starting point tailored for you in this ego death guide. Uncovering these aspects not only unveils the starting point for your transformative journey but also sheds light on elements within your life, self, and emotions that may interfere with your ability to be unconditionally free (even during your trips). Simply scratching the surface of these elements allows you to channel your energy effectively during your journeys. However, the aim is to empower you without overwhelming your emotions. Now is the opportune moment to gain a gentle understanding of yourself.

Consider capturing the flow of your thoughts by jotting down your answers in a notebook or on a separate piece of paper—a simple yet powerful way to navigate the labyrinth of your mind.

INNER DIALOGUE: YOUR INNER TRUTHS

1. Where am I in life? What has brought me to this moment of self-development? (Describe how you got here.)

2. How much do I understand myself, my actions, and my behaviors? (Describe what you understand so far.)

3. Do I have a lot of missing memories or blanks in my story? (Describe two or three emotionally impactful parts of your story that you have clarity on.)

4. In what ways do I struggle with being the person I feel I can be, the authentic me?

5. Is spacing out, procrastination, or short bursts of depression normal for me? (Describe how you use your energy, or where you focus it.)

6. Is my past something I feel comfortable discussing, even with myself?

These questions mark the beginning of your exploration. After answering these questions, I hope you have a clearer understanding of yourself, even if it's simply a broad understanding. Embracing your journey entails acknowledging that avoidance of heavy emotions is a natural defense mechanism. Be gentle with yourself and tune in to the subtle language your body speaks. Are you tense? Do you have any unexplainable pains or sensations, especially in the chest and back areas? Do your thoughts go blank when feeling the pressure of searching for answers? How's your jaw or throat? Observing these cues marks the beginning of a patient and compassionate journey toward self-awareness.

If you sense any tension, it could be a clue to the intensity of your emotions. If these questions have felt like a walk in the park, kudos! Your answers serve as a guide, setting the tone for the path you're already navigating. While this exploration may mark a new beginning, your past shapes the landscape behind you. You'll be building upon the foundations life has laid so far.

Now that you've set the right headspace, let's dive into self-analysis to pinpoint where you want to focus your attention. This journey is about understanding yourself deeply and choosing the paths that resonate most with your current state. With this self-analysis, your aim is to gain clarity on which psychedelic experience aligns best with your unique journey.

PSYCHEDELIC EXPLORATION 101

Feeling disconnected is a shared human experience, and your psychedelic journey can be a profound exploration of the parts within yourself that may be unaligned. Let's break down the subtleties of disconnection, diving into how we recognize its presence and grasping its impact on our journey toward liberation.

First, what does it mean to be disconnected? It implies there's something to connect to, a subtle awareness that might have been overlooked or, at times, consciously ignored. It's a common sensation that holds more meaning than we might realize.

Navigating through the complexities of the physical world, you might find yourself pulled in various directions, gradually distancing from the starting point of your life's journey. The feeling of disconnection is a by-product of the countless external experiences and influences shaping our existence.

So, how do you recognize if you're experiencing disconnection? Here are some general indicators that shed light on what it's like to be disconnected from your mind, body, soul/spirit, or perhaps all of the above.

WHAT IS MENTAL DISCONNECTION?

Being disconnected from your mind is essentially being out of touch with your intuition, that subtle inner guidance. This disconnection often stems from the noise of external influences, lingering echoes of past experiences, or the subtle yet powerful murmurs of your subconscious thoughts, steering your decisions and actions.

Recognizing this disconnection from your mind might not be straightforward, but it typically manifests in various ways. You may find yourself in a state of depression, confusion, caught in the monotony of repetitive loops, or living life on autopilot. It surfaces when you're living life inauthentically, concealing your true thoughts and emotions, or acting out narratives that lack emotional authenticity. The signs are evident when you start making excuses for things you don't genuinely want in your life, grappling with unresolved problems, enduring unhealthy relationships, feeling trapped in your circumstances, and facing inexplicable difficulties. The weight of anxiety, guilt, and perpetual fatigue becomes a familiar companion—these could be echoes of a mind seeking reconnection.

WHAT IS BODY DISCONNECTION?

Being disconnected from your body is essentially being estranged from your heart, the core of your emotional self. This disconnection reflects in how you treat both yourself and others, shaping patterns that influence what you attract into and out of your life. Your perspective on self-love, the significance of love in your life, and any underlying fears of love and happiness are all intertwined in this complex web.

This subtle disconnection casts a shadow over your thoughts and feelings, veiling them in a hint of darkness. It may manifest in closed-off attitudes, making it challenging to embrace new experiences and expand your horizons. The disconnect from the heart can induce a sense of paralysis and stagnation in the flow of life, leading to recurring mistakes and self-sabotage. Feeling disconnected from the heart might have become so ingrained that you're oblivious to the deeper reasons behind recurring patterns. It forms a distorted lens through which you view yourself and life, creating a normalcy around these disconnections.

WHAT IS SPIRITUAL DISCONNECTION?

Being disconnected from your spiritual self is, in essence, an intense connection to the ego self, a tether to the material and immediate aspects of existence.

Various factors contribute to this disconnection, ranging from unawareness of your spiritual self to inherited beliefs, repressed anger, and a distracted mindset overwhelmed by the chaos of the physical world.

Detecting spiritual disconnection can be challenging, sharing commonalities with disconnections from the mind and body. However, what sets it apart is an unexplainable loneliness or emptiness within, a void that seems impossible to fill. You might perceive yourself as a victim of life and your circumstances, grappling with a sense of powerlessness, accompanied by the weight of worrying and fear. This disconnection may manifest in dismissing certain aspects of your life, creating a gap between your spiritual self and the unfolding reality. In this state, you might find solace in satisfying physical needs, yet dismiss the importance of your overall physical and emotional health. The spiritual disconnection intertwines with the complexities of the mind and heart, creating a unique blend of difficulties that can be challenging to discern.

Have you found resonance with any of these mind, body, or spirit disconnections? Take your time to reflect, perhaps during meditation or before drifting into sleep tonight. Recognizing the disconnections within yourself is the initial stride toward reconnection, setting you on the trajectory for realignment. In the forthcoming steps of this manual, you'll be guided through a deliberate psychedelic journey aimed at reconnecting with these facets of yourself. The unique power of psychedelics lies in their ability to offer tangible insights into the metaphysical and abstract realms of life. This, in turn, renders our expedition toward emotional, spiritual, and mental elevation more accessible and comprehensible.

...SO, PSILOCYBIN, LSD, OR AYAHUASCA?

Now that we've laid the groundwork for your journey, let's explore the distinctive paths that lie ahead. Each option is a remarkable path to explore, with its own unique characteristics.

Magic mushrooms, naturally occurring in various parts of the world, present a connection to the Earth's cycles. These fungi contain the hallucinogenic compounds psilocybin and psilocin. From the enchanting appearance of wild varieties to the handcrafted versions cultivated for specific experiences, these fungi have a rich history. Psilocybin mushrooms can be ingested by simply chewing and swallowing or incorporating into teas and foods (dried or fresh). If you find yourself adrift, feel disconnected from your true self, and intuitively sense that there's more to your existence, psilocybin offers a gentle guide. It's for the souls who crave profound change and are yearning for clarity, a path to realign thoughts, emotions, and actions.

LSD, also known as lysergic acid diethylamide, is a synthetic compound derived from ergot fungus. Its production involves precise laboratory processes, and it was first synthesized by Swiss chemist Albert Hofmann in 1938. LSD is often consumed in small paper squares known as blotter paper, typically taken orally by allowing it to dissolve under the tongue or swallowing for digestion. For those sensing the weight of the world on their shoulders, craving a wake-up call to their divine purpose, LSD will show you the way to your reality and what you can make of it. This is for the souls who need to awaken to the boundless possibilities that await, allowing you to redefine your narrative and explore the limitless horizons of your capabilities.

Ayahuasca, an herbal brew prepared from a combination of Amazonian plants, beckons with ancient shamanic traditions using the *Banisteriopsis caapi* vine and *Psychotria viridis* leaves, skillfully blended to form a ceremonial potion. Traditionally, it is consumed in ceremonial settings under the guidance of experienced practitioners. If you carry deep emotional wounds or feel an unsettling disconnection from your own soul, this is a journey to begin with. For the wounded soul seeking an enriched calling from the universe, ayahuasca can allow for a profound recognition that your mind and body are powerful tools in the design of life. Ayahuasca is the sacred medicine offering a path to mend the fractures, connecting the dots between your emotional world and your soul's journey.

MY EXPERT PERSPECTIVE ON PSYCHEDELIC ROUTES

Every journey is a distinct adventure, and even when taking the same substance multiple times, the experience can vary. This highlights the significance of your inner self—your mind and emotions. Selecting an option based solely on comfort might not be the most beneficial decision. Instead, consider what aligns best with your current circumstances on this journey.

By now, you've gained a deeper understanding of yourself and developed a more personal connection with these psychedelics, grasping what each has to offer on an intimate level. Now, let me share what I've learned over the years, offering insights from guiding many on their journeys and from my own personal experiences.

When it comes to finding liberation, healing, and attaining clarity to elevate the mindset, my go-to recommendation is always psilocybin mushrooms. Yet, LSD has played a significant role in my growth and became the key that opened doors within my mind. It became my tool for liberating my mind from the constraints of my established personality and perception. During the beginning of my journey, I found the need to rewire my brain, reconnect with my mind, and rediscover the essence of who I was and who I aspired to become. On the other hand, mushrooms have been a true gift, providing a gentle guide through the twists and turns of the human experience. These incredible fungi helped create a harmonious rhythm between my thoughts and emotions, allowing for a more accessible journey into self-discovery. Importantly, they've offered a unique lens to explore and understand my body, fostering a profound connection with how I experience myself within this world.

Through my experiences with helping others on their journeys, I've realized that some individuals truly need to engage with their spirits first and foremost. Their emotions, life stories, and current circumstances might pose challenges in connecting with their mind and heart. I've come to understand that the disconnections people carry significantly influence the paths they should explore with these psychedelics. Consider someone who has long been disconnected from both the heart and mind; diving into the vast realm of the mind without a clear understanding of themself can be overwhelming. The intensity of feeling so alive during the experience may create a stark contrast with their daily life, leading to distraction. On the other hand, individuals who have endured emotional trauma or carry negative experiences often require a sense of liberation.

Many people regularly carry a weight that completely disconnects them from their higher selves. While the experience of elevation is incredible and freeing, bridging these aspects of themselves can be challenging, leading to a sense of dissociation.

In such cases, a spiritual reconnection becomes essential to harmonize these distinct parts of the self. So, the choice of whether to begin the awakening from the heart, mind, or spirit becomes a crucial consideration based on your unique journey.

I recommend using LSD and psilocybin for your ego death journey due to their profound abilities to unlock deep parts of your mind and soul. However, I also include ayahuasca for those who may feel extremely detached from their inner selves. It's possible to become so accustomed to this detachment that naturally flowing with the rhythm of your mind and soul becomes challenging. Ayahuasca offers an experience that makes the relationship between your body and soul more vulnerable and receptive, allowing you to open up more easily.

LSD and psilocybin can grant access to various dimensions of your consciousness, but if you dissociate from your body, the experience might not reach the depth needed for effective change. The goal is to have all aspects of yourself—mind, body, and soul—undergo the same transformative experience. This unity ensures that you can embody the sense of liberation and fluidity in your day-to-day life. By integrating the insights and revelations from these journeys, you can navigate life with a renewed sense of purpose and clarity, bringing harmony to your entire being.

To aid you in making an informed choice, I've crafted a chart that allows you to discern what resonates most with you. Trust your intuition, as you inherently know what's best for you and what you need most on this transformative journey.

If you decide to start with ayahuasca, recognize that this is a beautiful and significant first step in reconnecting with your spirit. However, this reconnection is only the beginning. The next essential steps involve reconnecting with your mind and heart. For this, I recommend exploring psilocybin to experience a Level 1 ego death. This transformative process will help strip away the mental barriers that hinder true freedom and excellence. By peeling back these layers, you'll release attachments to aspects of your life that hold you back, breaking through limitations and unlocking your full human potential.

PSYCHEDELIC JOURNEY NAVIGATOR

CRITERIA	PSILOCYBIN	LSD	AYAHUASCA
MINDSET & AWARENESS	Ideal for introspection and self-reflection	Best suited for enhancing creativity and cognitive exploration	Well-suited for deep emotional healing and spiritual awakening
EMOTIONAL LANDSCAPE	Effective for addressing anxiety, depression, and body disconnection with emotional clarity	Can promote emotional resilience and openness, leading to a spark of emotional revelations	Known for addressing trauma and fostering emotional release
SPIRITUAL CONNECTION	May enhance a sense of spiritual connectedness to one's self and the vibrational surroundings	Can induce profound and various spiritual experiences, unveiling the boundless dimensions of your spiritual self	Renowned for facilitating spiritual awakening and connection
SETTING & ENVIRONMENT	Well-suited for both solitary and group experiences	Versatile, adaptable to various settings, but often preferred in controlled environments	Traditionally experienced in ceremonial settings with a shamanic guide
DURATION OF EXPERIENCE	Moderate duration, typically 4–6 hours	Longer duration, ranging from 8–12 hours	Various durations, ranging from 4–8 hours, depending on the brew's strength
RECOMMENDED STARTING POINT	Well-suited for beginners exploring psychedelics, occking a balance between introspection and emotional well-being	Ideal for those familiar with psychedelics looking to deepen spiritual and consciousness exploration	Recommended for individuals seeking profound emotional healing and a deep dive into spiritual realms

MICRODOSING VS. FULL DOSES

Microdosing and using higher doses of psychedelics offer vastly different experiences, each with its unique benefits and limitations. Microdosing, typically involving around 0.1 to 0.3 grams of psilocybin mushrooms or a fraction of an LSD tab (about 10 to 20 micrograms), can provide a subtle yet profound shift in mindset. It allows you to connect more easily with your inner self and experience a heightened sense of clarity and creativity. This gentle approach helps you maintain your daily routines while enjoying an enhanced perception of your surroundings.

However, the reason microdosing falls short for achieving a proper ego death is that it allows you to hold on to your ego. Your sense of self, which acts as an anchor, remains intact. This anchor keeps you tethered to your familiar ways of thinking, feeling, and being, making it difficult to let go and flow freely into the unknown. To truly experience an ego death, you need to feel a sense of becoming nothing, just pure consciousness detached from your body. This separation from your ego, even for a moment, can lead to profound liberation and transformation.

Achieving an ego death typically requires a more substantial dose—around 3.5 grams (an eighth) of psilocybin mushrooms or a full tab of LSD (100 to 200 micrograms). At these higher doses, you are more likely to experience a profound shift in consciousness that allows you to detach from your ego. The first layer of ego death involves recognizing that your consciousness is not merely attached to your human body; instead, you are a consciousness that temporarily inhabits a body. This reversal of perception is essential. You must first accept your human existence and deeply understand what it truly means to be human.

While microdosing allows your mind to operate within its usual structures, albeit with an enhanced perspective, a full dose compels you to confront the vastness of your consciousness beyond the confines of your physical form. This deeper exploration is necessary for true ego dissolution, as it dismantles the structured ways of thinking and being that you unknowingly cling to, ultimately allowing for profound and lasting transformation.

✳ ☽ ✳

CHAPTER 6

PREPARING FOR THE JOURNEY

Whether you've had psychedelic experiences before or are venturing into this realm for the first time, preparing for your ego death journey will require mindfulness, intellect, and inner strength. There are two ways to navigate your existence: with intention or by default. As you experience the transformative effects of psychedelics, you must choose to either take control of your journey or let it control you.

One crucial aspect to address is the concept of "bad trips" and how to avoid them.

WHAT IS A BAD TRIP & HOW CAN YOU AVOID ONE?

Bad trips, much like euphoric trips, vary from person to person. What one considers a bad trip might not seem so terrible to someone else. This is because bad trips are deeply connected to the individual's thought patterns and emotional energy.

In everyday life, we have the ability to direct our focus wherever we want, often using distractions to avoid uncomfortable feelings or thoughts. We can easily divert our attention with activities, social interactions, or even substances to numb any pain. However, when on psychedelics, this ability is significantly diminished. Instead of just being, you are fully immersed in experiencing your reality, which requires much more effort to navigate your mind.

The best way to describe a bad trip is when you are overwhelmed by negative thoughts or emotions and lose the ability to steer your experience. Psychedelics amplify your inner world, bringing it to life in a deep, abstract, and tangible way, forcing you to confront these negative parts of your existence head-on. If you're not feeling well, that becomes your truth, along with the reasons behind those feelings.

On psychedelics, your mind experiences the unfiltered reality of your emotions and thoughts. The key to understanding this is recognizing that we have full dominion over our experiences. Although everything may seem out of control during a bad trip, trying to resist negative energy, emotions, and vibrations only intensifies them. If you immerse yourself in fear, your reality will mirror that energy, creating a cycle that perpetuates until you actively choose to stop it. The more you fight against these negative emotions, the more you expand and elongate the experience, falling deeper into the emotions it brings.

This amplified state of mind requires a different approach: one of acceptance and understanding. When things don't feel pleasant, your instinct shouldn't be to run away. Instead, approach every sensation with curiosity and bravery. It takes courage and stillness to dissect the language of your vibrations.

By acknowledging and addressing these feelings rather than avoiding them, you can transform your experience from one of fear and discomfort to one of insight and healing. The journey involves navigating these intense emotions with the awareness that they are temporary and a part of your deeper self that seeks resolution and integration.

GAINING CONTROL OVER YOUR PSYCHEDELIC EXPERIENCE

Embarking on a psychedelic journey is a profound endeavor that requires thoughtful preparation to ensure a safe, insightful, and meaningful experience. When I talk about gaining control over your trip, I'm not referring to rigid limiting or suppressing the experience. Instead, it's about being mindful and intentionally preparing so that you can navigate the journey with awareness and purpose. This type of control allows you to create a space for a deep dive into your psyche while ensuring a safe and profound experience that can add value to your life. Here are the key steps to prepare yourself for this sacred experience:

1. Treat the experience as sacred.

First and foremost, recognize that this journey is sacred. The mindset with which you approach your trip will significantly influence its outcome. This is not just another recreational activity; it's a deep dive into your entire existence, offering you the opportunity to access aspects of life that may otherwise seem impossible or divine. Approach your experience with reverence and respect, understanding that you are engaging with a powerful tool for transformation. Treating your journey as sacred helps set a tone of mindfulness, ensuring that you are open to the insights and changes that may come.

2. Understand the importance of energy.

Energy is a fundamental aspect of a successful psychedelic journey. The energy in your environment, the energy of the people around you, and your own energy all play crucial roles. You want to flow naturally, and any external energy could potentially interrupt this flow. This is why it's essential to have complete control over the energy of your experience.

3. Choose your company wisely.

This journey is deeply personal and sacred, one that you should ideally undertake alone. The mind is an individual experience, and when aiming for an ego death, the journey inward is best navigated without external influences. Being alone allows you to fully concentrate on your inner world, helping you maintain the focus needed for a transformative experience. However, if you feel the need for extra support, having a trip sitter—a trusted companion who stays grounded and supports you during your journey—can be particularly valuable, especially if you're feeling uncertain about managing your mindset or navigating intense experiences. A trip sitter is typically helpful for those new to psychedelics, especially in moments when you may feel overwhelmed, and can provide peace of mind as well as help reduce the likelihood of a challenging or anxious experience.

That said, I find that the energy of others, no matter how trusted, can occasionally limit the full depth of self-exploration. In such a personal, intimate experience, even a well-intentioned sitter's presence can feel like a tether, subtly pulling you back from fully surrendering to the experience. This can be especially true when aiming to transcend the ego, as someone else's presence may unintentionally influence your emotional openness or limit your ability to explore deeply. If you feel a trip sitter would ease your journey, ensure that person is someone you can be 100 percent authentic with, someone you can discuss your intentions with, someone who respects the sanctity of this experience and brings a calm, supportive energy so you're both aligned on making this journey as open and safe as possible.

4. Create a safe and controlled environment.

Having full control over your environment is vital. This means finding a space where you can be alone and uninterrupted for an extended period. Even if you are tripping alone, make sure no one will waltz in and out of your space. Outside energies, no matter how well-meaning, can disrupt the natural flow of your thoughts and energy. Plan your trip for a time when you can ensure this solitude.

5. Prepare for vulnerability.

Be ready to embrace vulnerability. Understand that the process of ego death involves recognizing and dismantling the walls you've built to protect yourself from fear, pain, and discomfort. These walls are the constructs of your ego, which can be so subtle and abstract that they often go unnoticed. Even with the aid of psychedelics, your ego can skillfully disguise itself, maintaining its grip on you if you allow it.

The key is to first acknowledge that you have these defenses up. Once you recognize this, let your guard down and question why it was there in the first place. What are you protecting yourself from? By deeply exploring these questions, you can begin to understand the roots of your ego's defenses.

6. Set clear intentions.

Before beginning your journey, set clear intentions. This is a crucial step that will guide your experience and help you navigate through challenging moments. Knowing what you want to achieve, understand, or resolve can provide direction and meaning, making your trip more productive and insightful. Focus on being as open and as free as possible. Your goal should be to explore the vast capabilities of your mind and understand how it operates on different levels. Be prepared to encounter elevated parts of your mind as well as more mundane or challenging aspects. Recognize that everything presenting itself during your journey is significant and deserves your attention. Don't be passive about anything in your mind. Use these moments for true introspection and analyze yourself. Understand that the elements appearing between your higher purpose and your lower self exist within you all the time. If they are coming to the forefront during your psychedelic experience, it's for a reason. They are not to be ignored but explored and understood.

Additionally, consider recording your session with voice or video. This can be an invaluable tool to keep track of your experiences and insights, allowing you to reflect on them later. This documentation can help you make sense of your journey and integrate the lessons you have learned into your daily life.

7. Ground yourself.

Grounding techniques are essential for a balanced and insightful psychedelic journey. Grounding means creating a steady balance between your mind and body, which is crucial for gaining control over your experience. When your mind is focused on both your mental and physical states simultaneously, it anchors your energy under your control. This allows you to observe your thoughts and experiences rather than simply react to them, making it easier to flow with the effects of the psychedelics.

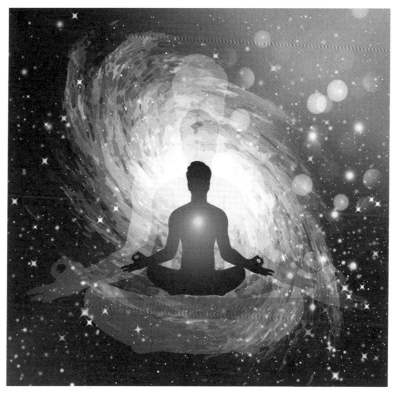

Grounding involves practices that help you connect with your body and the present moment. This can include meditation, deep breathing exercises, or light stretching. These activities center you, providing a solid foundation that makes it easier to manage and integrate the experiences you will have during your trip. Another effective grounding technique is listening to frequency music. This type of music can positively influence the tone of your environment. Choose frequencies that align with your intentions and feelings, such as love a frequency or god frequency, which you can easily find on YouTube. These frequencies can help create a positive and supportive atmosphere, enhancing your ability to stay grounded and focused.

By incorporating grounding techniques into your preparation, you'll create a solid foundation for your psychedelic journey.

8. Be open and accepting.

Approach your trip with an open and accepting mindset. Understand that you might encounter uncomfortable truths or challenging emotions. Accept these as part of the process. Resistance can create a negative feedback loop, exacerbating discomfort and fear. Instead, embrace whatever comes up with curiosity and compassion.

9. Eat lightly.

Finally, make sure to eat a couple of hours before starting your journey. During the experience, you might become so absorbed in the process that you forget about food. Keeping your body nourished beforehand will help ensure you feel comfortable and maintain your energy throughout.

By following these steps, you'll set the stage for a profound and transformative experience. Remember, this journey goes beyond the psychedelic substance itself; it's about exploring higher realms of your existence, accessing new dimensions of yourself, and navigating the intricate energies and vibrations of your surroundings with clarity and purpose.

RECOGNIZING THE EGO: WHAT TO EXPECT ON THE PATH TO EGO DEATH

Ego death is a profound journey, and before you can fully experience it, it helps to get familiar with the ego itself—the part of you that silently weaves through your thoughts, influencing your perceptions, reactions, and behaviors. You may have heard of the ego described as a mask or an illusion, but it's actually a bit more layered and elusive.

In your day-to-day life, the ego is like a character you've played for so long that it feels natural, almost invisible. It's the voice that steps in to affirm your choices, defend your opinions, and shape your sense of self. This "character" isn't only keeping things predictable—it's always working to uphold your comfort zone, whether that means reinforcing habits, thoughts, or even actions that don't necessarily align with your deeper truths. It might say things like, "You're doing fine; no need to change," or, "Better to play it safe." The ego character seems to support you, giving you a sense of continuity and safety, but it also limits your experience by subtly urging you to stay within familiar boundaries, even if that means ignoring what you genuinely want or feel.

Once you step into your psychedelic journey, the ego—crafted by years of conditioning and ingrained ideas about yourself—becomes strikingly visible. With the mind in a state of expanded awareness, you may start to see just how much of your thoughts, reactions, and view of reality have been shaped by this "invisible conductor." The ego is like a structure that has formed around your mind, a mental framework you've lived within for as long as you can remember. Because it's always been there, shaping how you see yourself and the world, it can feel as though you're naked without it. In moments like these, however, the ego's usual grip begins to loosen, and its once-solid ideas of "self" and "reality" feel as though they're melting away. As this layer dissolves, you're exposed to the raw and unfiltered dimensions of your own mind—your true character, your beliefs, your life, seen from a new, often startling perspective. In this openness, you're no longer bound by the ego's usual defenses; instead, you're free to observe yourself with an honesty that can be both illuminating and intense. This is the beginning of what's called an ego death—a process that's as liberating as it is humbling.

THE EXPERIENCE: SURRENDERING CONTROL AND RECOGNIZING YOURSELF

As you begin to feel the ego loosening, prepare yourself for a range of sensations some exhilarating, others unexpectedly resistant. While psychedelics can guide you to deeper layers of consciousness, it's essential to remember that you are still the one steering the journey. Your usual patterns, behaviors, and beliefs don't just vanish with the onset of the experience; instead, they may become more noticeable, even amplified, revealing how much of your perception and actions are guided by the ingrained habits and biases of the ego. This journey toward ego death is as intricate and unique as your own psyche. There's no one-size-fits-all path, no map to follow, no guarantee that psychedelics alone will carry you to this state. They can open doors to vast, hidden realms of your mind, but they won't automatically lead you through them. The real power—the potential for profound transformation—comes from within you. It's your willingness to confront, explore, and release the mind's familiar boundaries that will determine how far you go. This isn't something that happens to you; it's something you must actively engage with. Psychedelics may reveal what's possible, but the courage to dive in, to face what you find—that comes from you.

As you ease into this journey, you may find yourself moving through a paradox. Part of your mind senses an expansive openness, as if inner barriers are dissolving and you're free to observe life from a place beyond familiar limits. Yet, alongside this openness, there's often a subtle pull—a weight of resistance that tugs at you, urging you back to old, comfortable patterns of thought and behavior. This isn't just a mental or emotional resistance; it's the ego itself, sensing its hold loosening and trying to reassert its place in your perception of self.

The ego isn't "bad" for this; it's simply following its instinct to protect the sense of self it has upheld for so long. The challenge, and ultimately the beauty, lies in recognizing this push and pull and allowing yourself to sit with it—to observe the resistance without judgment or the need to control it.

It's not always easy, and it's certainly not automatic. Surrendering to this process is more like balancing on a fine line: it asks you to be present, to consciously let go of expectations, and to trust in the layers of insight waiting to emerge. By leaning into both the openness and the resistance, you'll find that ego death isn't a quick release or a sudden transformation, but a gradual unfolding of awareness that you guide, moment by moment.

EXPLORING YOUR MENTAL LANDSCAPE

During your psychedelic journey, you may start to notice how your thoughts move and connect. In many ways, this is how your mind has always worked, but with the veil lifted, it becomes easier to see. Thoughts don't just pop in and out of existence—they flow together, creating a web of ideas, memories, and beliefs that shape your perception. Think of it like a constellation, where each thought is a star, and the threads of association link them across the vastness of your consciousness. As you step into this space, you might see that some thoughts shine bright, demanding your attention, while others linger softly in the background, waiting for you to notice. These thought patterns are constantly in motion, sparking new associations and revealing the interconnected nature of your mental landscape.

What's important here is recognizing the flow. When you focus on how thoughts move—how they lead to one another, how they give birth to emotions or memories—you can begin to see the natural rhythm of your mind. This is the key to the experience: learning to flow with your thoughts, letting them come and go without interference. If there are buried thoughts or unaddressed emotions, they may try to surface. Don't rush to push them away or close them off; let them be.

As you observe this mental landscape, you gain a new sense of freedom. Some thoughts will feel vivid, demanding attention like bright stars in the night sky, while others remain faint, like distant galaxies in the periphery. By allowing your thoughts to emerge and flow freely, you unlock the true power of introspection. This is where the magic happens—when you let go of the instinctual need to "fix" or judge. Often, the ego jumps in, cutting off that flow, adding judgment, excuses, or distractions, trying to steer you away from deeper awareness. It might shift your focus, tell you "this isn't important," or

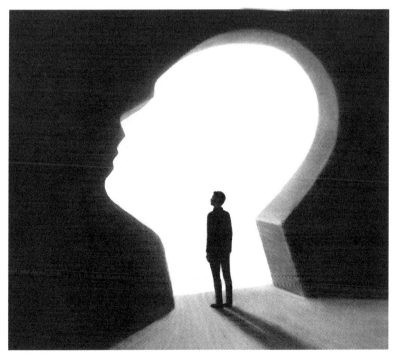

remind you of an old fear or belief that doesn't serve you anymore. These interruptions are the ego's way of maintaining control and keeping you stuck in predictable patterns.

ASK QUESTIONS TO FIND ANSWERS

One of the most transformative practices you can adopt in this state is the art of questioning. Asking "why" is deceptively simple yet incredibly potent. Why did that thought come up? Why do you suddenly feel this way? The key here is curiosity. It's not enough to notice things and think, "That's strange." Instead, dig deeper: Why is it showing up? What is it trying to reveal? This shift from passive observation to active questioning is what propels your introspection forward. Psychedelics may amplify the process, but it's your engagement—your willingness to inquire—that unlocks the true power of the experience. When you embrace curiosity, you allow your mind's natural flow to resume, and clarity begins to emerge from your thoughts and emotions. Questioning your reactions, feelings, and beliefs is how you regain mastery over your experience, enabling you to unearth the layers of truth that have been hidden in plain sight.

COMMUNICATION FROM THE SUBCONSCIOUS

As your mind opens, you may encounter vivid imagery, sensations, or scenarios that seem unfamiliar or unexpected.

This is your subconscious reaching out, using symbols and sensations to communicate truths that are difficult to capture in words. Normally, the ego holds tight boundaries around your conscious awareness, keeping the subconscious hidden. But in this state, as those boundaries soften, deeper parts of your psyche can begin to surface, especially emotions that may be tied to forgotten or unexpressed experiences. The subconscious can communicate in layers, revealing different facets of itself depending on where your awareness rests.

Instead of feeling disoriented or turning away, approach these messages with curiosity and openness. As you explore and accept what arises, you may begin to experience a shift in perspective, where your usual ways of thinking and perceiving begin to dissolve. The ego death process isn't simply about "losing" your sense of self; it's about untangling the dense web of beliefs, memories, and ideas that unknowingly define your sense of self, which is usually what holds you back. This unraveling might feel disorienting, even challenging, as it reveals perspectives you hadn't considered, but it also opens the door to see life with fresh eyes and from new angles.

A GRADUAL UNFOLDING

The journey of ego dissolution and self-reconnection is a multilayered process that unfolds gradually. It's important to approach this journey with patience and dedication, understanding that it may require several sessions to navigate through the various levels of your consciousness. Each layer of your consciousness holds a unique experience, and with the 1-3-2 method as your guide (see page 105), you can navigate this journey with clarity and focus. Next we'll explore various types of ego deaths, each unlocking a new level of awareness and connection with your true self.

CHAPTER 7

✳ ☽ ✳

LEVEL 1 EGO DEATH

Here, you will learn what it takes to achieve and what to expect from a Level 1 ego death, called such because it represents the culmination of your consciousness, integrating Levels 2 and 3. A Level 1 ego death embodies the wholeness of your being. It's common to feel deeply connected to a higher source and to sense a profound interconnectedness with everything in the universe while on psychedelics.

A Level 1 ego death is typically the first type of ego death people experience. This form of ego death is the easiest to encounter because the thought of our existence is always on the edge of our consciousness, even if we rarely bring it to the forefront. For those who feel that life is a burden, hard, or unfair, questioning why they exist, what would happen if they didn't exist, and why their life is the way it is causes their consciousness to dip in and out of awareness of their existence.

The reason this awareness remains on the edge rather than the forefront is that their perception is tuned into and focused on their problems rather than the entirety of their experience. They are unable to see themselves within their life stories and visualize the blank canvas ahead of them.

In reality, everything is about perception. Most people don't see the entirety of their existence—they only see what they are currently experiencing. The entirety of your experience includes seeing yourself within your life story, recognizing the blank canvas ahead of you, and understanding that anything is possible. It involves seeing your narrative, your character, your disadvantages and advantages, and your surroundings and comprehending the emotions you're experiencing so you know what you need. This broader perspective is difficult to achieve when our egos allow us to see only two steps ahead and continuously fill in future steps based on past experiences.

This is why the Level 1 ego death is so gracefully impactful. It shifts your perception from seeing life as a series of burdens to seeing it as a divine experience filled with potential. By embracing this awareness, you start to understand the power of your mind and the divine connection between your mind and body. This awareness centers on the simple fact that you are alive.

This kind of ego death is where the boundaries between your body, mind, and spirit begin to fade away. Many people go through life focused on just one part of their existence. In this state, you experience a beautiful unity of all dimensions of yourself. As your awareness grows, you stop feeling divided and instead become whole—rooted in your physical self, open in your thoughts, and connected to your spirit. It's in this integration that you discover the oneness that ties you to the very essence of life—complete and boundless.

STAGE 1: GROUNDING AND PREPARATION

The first step toward experiencing Level 1 ego death begins with selecting the right setting, ideally in nature. Being outdoors helps you tune into vibrations beyond your own, which can help your ego relax. And engaging all your senses awakens your mind to the present moment and attunes it to life's rhythms. But if you feel more comfortable at home, that space can also serve as a safe haven for your journey. Ultimately, it's about choosing the environment where you feel most relaxed, because the heart of this psychedelic experience resides in your mind, no matter where you are.

STAGE 2: ELEVATION & HEIGHTENED AWARENESS

Regardless of your location, focus is key. Whether you've chosen psilocybin or LSD, you'll begin to feel an elevation, whether in bodily sensations or heightened mental clarity. Although abstract, it feels as though your awareness is rising upward, almost as if shifting from the body to the mind. You can feel this shift slowly building as you become aware of subtle changes in your senses.

If your journey starts with physical sensations, you might notice gentle vibrations coursing through your body, especially in your fingers and hands. You may also feel a sense of weight in your chest, and your throat could feel more pronounced. These are key parts of your body that you constantly use and typically lose awareness of. During elevation, these parts become more noticeable.

Becoming physically conscious of your body as you experience the onset of the psychedelic can be overwhelming if you don't relax and stay in control. It's very important to trust yourself and consistently remember that this experience is about you—your mind, your energy, and your control of it all. The psychedelic substances are merely allowing you more access to what already exists within you.

Sit down in a comfortable position, take deep breaths, and with each breath in, mentally acknowledge that it is a breath in. With each breath out, acknowledge that it is a breath out. Continue this until you feel centered and become aware of the rise and fall of your chest. Saying and doing an action simultaneously keeps your mind and body in the same moment, helping you stay present.

It'll be easy to recognize when your mind begins elevating. You'll notice that your senses feel sharper; you'll see changes in the lighting or the color tone of your environment. Sometimes, a wave of euphoria or laughter just washes over you, like the sensation people experience at high altitudes or when taking in more oxygen. This happens because increased oxygen or changes in atmospheric pressure can lead to an altered state of consciousness, making the brain more sensitive and reactive. During the onset of psychedelics, a similar process occurs. Your brain chemistry changes, leading to heightened awareness and altered perceptions. This shift can feel like your mind is expanding, rising above your usual state of consciousness. Imagine your mind as a vast landscape, with new areas becoming illuminated and accessible. This elevation allows you to see and feel more, connecting deeply with your surroundings and your own internal experience.

Every person and every trip is different. Your conscious elevation could span anywhere between 30 minutes to two hours. How will you know when you are done elevating? By this point, you won't be too concerned about the elevation process itself; you will be so immersed in your experience that you will intuitively know the difference between the lower and higher selves. From this point forward, your psychedelic experience will be shaped entirely by you and your psyche. How you direct your energy will determine whether parts of your subconscious mind surface or whether you remain anchored in the present moment; understand that neither path is wrong.

What's been on your mind before you began your psychedelic journey may cause your subconscious to rise, and in these moments, allow it to. But remember to stay in control—be curious and try to understand what your inner self is trying to communicate and why. If you encounter "trippy" sensations, I encourage you to maintain your mental and physical control, using your power to gently redirect your focus toward the present moment by simply breathing.

For instance, during moments when you may perceive trippy visuals or sensations of movement around you, resist the urge to be entertained by them. If you notice vibrational waves around your environment, this may signify that your reality is clashing with your emotions. Although it may appear surreal, take a moment to reflect on what you are feeling and what might have triggered these emotions. This introspection is key. Observe everything within yourself and your surroundings. The more you question, the more your mind will expand.

During this phase of your psychedelic journey, keep your eyes open and fixate on something that captures your attention, preferably the Level 1 ego psychedelic image provided at the end of this chapter. This image serves as a reminder of the ego placed around your mind, blocking a seamless connection with the universe.

STAGE 3: CONFRONTING THE EGO

LIFE & DEATH

As mentioned earlier in this book, your first level of ego death is acknowledging that you are human, alive, and inevitably, one day, you will die. These are the simple facts of our existence, but we rarely pay attention to them. Many people find the topic of death uncomfortably morbid, but this avoidance stems from a disconnection between the mind and our existence.

In everyday life, it's easy to get caught up in the surface—your routine, responsibilities, and character—focusing on the details while avoiding the bigger questions of life. We often take for granted the amazing things our bodies do—every heartbeat, each breath, the flow of blood—forgetting how precious our time is. This disconnection from ourselves starts early, shaped by the way we're taught and the influences around us. Whether through religion, culture, or upbringing, we are given certain perspectives on life and death. Without a deep understanding of the mind's power and the spiritual experiences it can offer, your connection to life may not be as strong as your fear of death.

It's easy to push thoughts of death to the back of your mind, avoiding the discomfort they bring. But on psychedelics, this awareness becomes impossible to ignore. The balance between life and death is no longer abstract—it's felt in every breath and heartbeat. You become keenly aware of the life force within you, the energy that animates your body, and with it, the fragile line that separates existence from nothingness.

This heightened awareness creates a deep appreciation for simply being alive, turning fear of death into gratitude for life. In a single, conscious moment during your psychedelic experience, you may realize something profound: you are a spiritual being temporarily inhabiting a physical body. This is more of a privilege than a burden. Think about how often you get caught up in the stress of responsibilities and forget that simply being alive is a gift. This gift gives you the opportunity to feel, see, taste, and hear all the beauty this world has to offer. Yes, life comes with its challenges, but those pressures don't define our existence. Too often, we allow the weight of our circumstances to cloud the simple truth: we are an energetic being, given the opportunity to experience existence.

What your ego self faces during this part of your journey is that what actually defines your existence is how you choose to experience life. You are an infinite energy living through this unique avatar, shaped by the time, place, and circumstances you were born into. Even the positioning of the stars and planets at your birth influences the flow of your energy. Your genetics, upbringing, and story create a one-of-a-kind perspective—a way for this energy to witness the world in a way only you can. Every detail—big or small—is a chance for this energy to experience, learn, and appreciate the beauty of simply being alive. There are many layers to how this energy perceives reality. When we're stuck in our lower-dimensional self, viewing life through just one limited lens, it keeps us from seeing the meaning and endless possibilities life has to offer.

This energy that flows within you is life itself. The circumstances and details of your story are simply the backdrop to the deeper experience of living. No matter the path, life offers countless opportunities to embrace its beauty if you're willing to listen. And one of the most important ways to do that is by understanding the language of your emotions, rather than being swept away by them.

Think about when your heart races with fear, that immense power at work within you is the same power that allows you to feel joy. When emotions are entangled with the ego, especially emotional pain, they tend to dominate our reality, making it natural to try to control what we feel—or don't feel. That divine energy becomes restricted, held captive by the ego instead of flowing freely, preventing us from truly experiencing and understanding the lessons our emotions have to offer. Imagine for a moment that, in death, this divine energy—the very essence of life—will cease to exist. During this journey, you'll recognize that both the highs and lows of your emotional experience are simply two sides of the same coin. Your perception shapes how you navigate this energy, and embracing it fully allows you to truly savor all that life has to offer. After all, feeling the intensity of life is far more enriching than confronting the emptiness of nothingness.

LINEAR VS. CYCLICAL TIME

By the time you are deep into your journey, your sense of time will have disappeared, leading to an enlightening realization that time doesn't exactly exist in the first place. It's merely a structured way of living based on our systematic world. Our sense of time isn't something random we've made up—it mirrors the design of our universe. We base it on the natural order of day and night, the cycle of the sun and the moon. However, because human lives are brief compared to the vast timeline of the universe, we tend to think in smaller increments of time. We break it down from hour to hour, day to day, week to week, month to month, year to year, and everything in between becomes the specific details of our lives.

Our ego is heavily dependent on this sense of time, creating a frame or box around our minds that traps the thoughts that eventually turn our minds into a maze. The concept of structure is an essential aspect of our reality, deeply rooted in the nature of the universe. However, the key difference between humanity and the universe lies in our emotional connection to time—we feel stress, doubt, worry, and fear, and these feelings are tied to a linear perspective. The universe doesn't experience time like an hourglass, with moments slipping away. Instead, it operates on a cyclical system, where time is a continuous loop rather than a linear path. This cyclical structure solidifies the truth that everything existing in the moment is interconnected, with each event being a cause and effect of the next. The universe is beautifully organized, ensuring that every moment and action flows effortlessly into the bigger picture of existence.

This level of ego death reveals a profound truth: our human experience, with all its complexities, is just a reflection of the universe's dual nature. Our journey through this unique existence is shaped by both our mind and heart. This duality functions like a pedal and a steering wheel—one providing power, the other offering direction, propelling us through life with purpose and clarity.

Just as the universe flows through its cycles, we too flow between these states, shaped by the rhythms of day and night. During the day, when the sun is up, we tend to think with more structure and logic. The sun's energy pushes our decisions to be calculated and rational. But when night falls and the moon rises, we are drawn inward. Our emotional side surfaces, and we become more introspective, vulnerable, and reflective. This is when we let ourselves feel fully, and we tend to make decisions based on emotion rather than reason.

This cyclical shift between logic and emotion is natural, but many people lean too heavily on one side or the other or even shift between the two. They might choose logic during the day when it suits their need for control, and emotions at night when they feel more vulnerable. While both perspectives are valid and important parts of who you are, relying on one while neglecting the other creates imbalance. True alignment comes when you consciously integrate these two sides—merging your logical, action-oriented self with your emotional, reflective self.

Now, the ego isn't just hidden in your logic during the day; it quietly dictates your thoughts and decisions, whether you're acting logically or emotionally, influencing both realms in ways you may not realize. To truly understand the transformative power of this Level 1 ego death experience, you must first recognize how the distinction between linear and cyclical time impacts the way you live, think, and create your reality.

Linear time tends to trap us in reactive habits, where subconscious thoughts, unresolved emotions, and past events quietly guide our choices. This mode leads us to unknowingly manifest a life that doesn't align with our true desires or potential. We can get stuck in a routine, reacting to old wounds, frustrations, or fears without realizing they're shaping our present and future.

In contrast, cyclical time offers a more expansive, conscious way of experiencing life. Cyclical time allows you to see life as a web of possibilities. With this broader perspective, you'll notice how emotions and situations come back around, giving you the chance to use your journey to empower your future. Here, you have the power to use both your emotions and logic as complementary forces. Rather than reacting, you begin to steer your life intentionally, creating a reality based on your current desires and deeper truths.

What makes life so unknowingly challenging is how easily we fall into linear thinking, keeping our focus narrow and fixed on our daily priorities. We often get so committed to the version of ourselves we present to the world (our persona) that we only allow certain thoughts to surface, mainly those aligned with immediate concerns like financial security, career success, or meeting desires. When we let our ego take charge, we tend to focus on what feels urgent, leaving those deeper emotional thoughts waiting for our attention. For example, work life can occupy a significant amount of your time and mental space, and because it's tied to your livelihood, you convincingly believe it to be your top priority. But this can distract you from other important aspects of your life, such as emotional well-being or even personal passions. Also, when the primal urges of the id blend with the ego's justifications, we can find ourselves making impulsive decisions that ignore our deeper emotions and true desires. This usually leads us to prioritize immediate desires over meaningful connections, leaving our emotional needs unfulfilled.

We often let our egos dominate our decisions, which creates a disconnect between our true selves and our perceived reality— which means these ego-driven thoughts present only a partial view of who we truly are. Beyond the version of ourselves that we project out into the world, there exist other versions that we don't present to the world, or sometimes even to ourselves.

As the ego stands in the way of the entirety of your inner self, you remain blind to the entirety of your reality. True self-awareness means embracing all aspects of your psyche, even those thoughts lingering on the edge of your consciousness, semi-visible yet influential. These thoughts, if left unexamined, can deceive you into believing they do not exist at all. Recognizing and understanding the patterns of your thought processes is pivotal in gaining genuine control over your reality. Through your psychedelic journey, you have the chance to explore these deeper thoughts, paying close attention to how they've influenced your past actions and shaped your current reality.

STAGE 4: DISMANTLING THE EGO

Understanding life, death, and time on an intellectual level is one thing, but truly experiencing them on a conscious level is something else entirely. Without breaking through the ego, these thoughts can feel like abstract philosophical musings—easy to comprehend, but hard to truly absorb. Psychedelics shift your mind in a way that allows you to consciously experience life and time outside of your habitual, linear thought process. You no longer just contemplate these truths—you live them.

When your psychedelics begin to kick in, they ease a part of your mind called the default mode network, which is responsible for several parts of your cognitive functioning, but this is basically the part of your brain that anchors you to your current sense of self and reality. It's like your mind trapped within a box made of your routine thoughts, fears, and defenses. What makes psychedelics a mind- and life-altering experience is that they make you feel as though this mental box vanishes, and suddenly, every part of your mind—your emotions, logic, and core truths—are able to move freely together. In this expanded state, the surface-level, ego-driven self that you normally identify with is seen for what it is—a barrier that restricts your whole self.

Think back to the layers of existence we explored earlier. Remember that the outer tier is spiritual and non-physical, a space where reality becomes more abstract and moves beyond what's simply tangible. As we move inward, our experience of life becomes more concrete and personal. At the very center of this tiered existence lies the ego—the sense of self that anchors you to the physical world and your identity. Although I've described the ego as a barrier, it does serve a purpose—it keeps your consciousness anchored in the tangible world. However, the problems arise when the ego goes beyond its role, not just anchoring your existence, but also dividing and controlling your thoughts and emotions.

This particular ego death process isn't about discarding the ego entirely but about loosening its grip, allowing your consciousness to flow freely through those multilevel tiers of existence. As the ego's grip continues to ease, something truly significant happens: your emotional self (Level 2 consciousness) and higher self (Level 3 consciousness) come together, allowing you to consciously experience your thoughts and emotions as a unified, cohesive stream of awareness. Flowing with these unified senses of thought allows you to understand both yourself and life with remarkable clarity, where your inner world moves in perfect harmony with your outer reality. In this state, the division between "self" and "reality" dissolves. You aren't just observing your life; you're fully immersed in it, effortlessly navigating both your inner emotional world and the external world around you. This fusion allows you to experience life as a continuous, connected stream, where you move through each moment fully present and deeply aligned.

This stage is about reclaiming your power by realizing that you are the architect of your reality. When you let go of the ego, the energy within and around you aligns your physical self, mind, and spirit, merging your thoughts, feelings, and intentions into a seamless experience of reality. True liberation lies in this balance—understanding that neither your past nor external forces dictate your future, but the alignment of your inner self, consciousness, and reality does. This is the true meaning of becoming "one."

PSYCHEDELIC MILESTONES

Bookmark the following page and keep it open before you consume your psychedelic substance. During your trip, reading long passages may feel overwhelming, so use this milestone to help you focus on achieving your ego death and becoming "one."

PSYCHEDELIC MILESTONES

Level 1 Ego Death

Remove the box from around your mind.

Open to the universe.

Your Mind + Your Heart
+ Your Actions
– One (Whole)

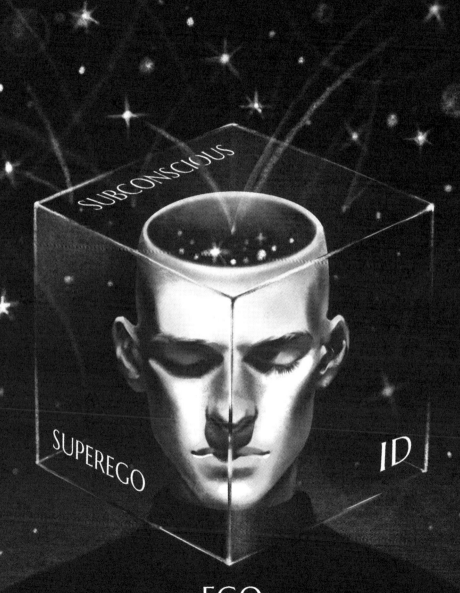

CHAPTER 8

✳ ☽ ✳

LEVEL 3 EGO DEATH: THE THIRD-EYE AWAKENING

Welcome to the next stage of your journey: Level 3 ego death, a deep dive into the inner workings of your existence. This is where your mental consciousness reaches new heights, where your third eye awakens, and where the true essence of your being is unveiled. At this stage, the boundaries of ordinary perception dissolve, allowing you to experience your mind in extraordinary ways. Encountering a third-eye awakening on psychedelics is actually quite common, yet it holds a unique power that many fail to fully harness.

Many who explore psychedelics see it as an escape—a chance to step out of their everyday reality, experience an altered state of mind, and view their trip as a temporary break from the mundane, believing they will simply "return to normal" once the effects wear off. What they may not realize is that this outlook subtly determines their commitment to a life of dissatisfaction and unrealized potential. The true essence of using psychedelics lies in understanding how to maintain a heightened, open, and expanded state of mind continually— not merely as a brief departure, but as a pathway to sustained bliss, health, and multidimensional success. This perception is a subtle choice, one that depends heavily on your mindset, intention, and willpower.

When I experienced my first trips on psilocybin and LSD, my initial reaction was not to escape but to understand. I was captivated by how my mind could function so differently. I questioned everything: why my thoughts were clearer, how my senses were heightened, and how my inner dialogue seemed so much denser and more immediate. As I dove deeper into my psychedelic experience, I realized that my brain isn't just a brain, it's a sophisticated machine, operating with a delicate and intricate design. This machine not only processes vast amounts of information but also channels a seamless flow of energy throughout its mechanical space. I realized that the energy I was experiencing was my mind itself. It may sound simple, but really think about it: What is a mind? What is this energy coursing through our consciousness? Where does it come from, and what is it made of? The mind is an intricate network of thoughts, emotions, and perceptions, all driven by this unseen yet powerful energy. This realization pushed me to contemplate the very essence of consciousness and the incredible design that allows us to experience reality.

As I moved through my environment, I realized that my brain was also simultaneously managing countless tasks. It was recognizing new and familiar surroundings, observing my movements, coordinating my body's functions, and allowing me to think about all of these processes—and much more—with astonishing speed. My thoughts were traveling at the speed of light, allowing me to witness and contemplate everything simultaneously. The psychedelics didn't transform my mind's capabilities; they simply allowed me to observe its true nature. In this heightened state of awareness, I saw the true complexity and brilliance of human design.

It was then that I realized the power of choice in these psychedelic experiences. With curiosity and courage, I chose to look behind the curtains of reality and explore the deeper dimensions of consciousness. Many people, intimidated by the vastness of existence, confine their conscious experience to the physical level. When faced with the boundless expanses of the mind, some individuals unknowingly grasp onto their egos for stability, clinging to what they perceive as their identity and sense of self.

During this ego death, releasing the constraints of your ego reveals the inner mechanics of your mind. This deeper awareness shows you how you truly operate, offering insights into the control you have over your avatar—your body and mind—and transforming how you experience reality and your place within it. It's the soul, not the ego, that guides us to explore beyond the surface, unlocking the deeper potential of our lives.

STAGE 1: GROUNDING AND PREPARATION

For a Level 3 ego death, your environment might differ from that of Level 1. While nature is beneficial, I recommend staying home for this deeply internal journey. It requires intense mental focus and detachment from your physical body. Find a quiet place to sit still and focus on your breath. Feel the rhythm of your chest rising and falling with each breath, and continue to narrate your experiences even as the effects of the psychedelics take hold and elevate your awareness. Whatever sensations you experience within your body due to the elevation from the psychedelics, allow your mind to become aware of them. This mindful focus helps you maintain balance and control between your mind and body throughout the experience.

This part of the ego death process is simple but crucial—it's where you cross the threshold from experiencing to observing. Pay close attention to the voice in your mind that narrates your actions.

During meditation, focusing solely on the present moment can be challenging because the mind is easily distracted by passing thoughts. Experiencing stillness for more than a few minutes takes practice, and as you learn the effort it requires, you'll notice how many thoughts can race through your mind in seconds. However, on psychedelics, you may find greater control over this mental stability, especially when you focus on your breathing. Narrating your actions as you do them helps your mind and body sync in the present moment.

If your thoughts begin to wander, that's okay. Your goal is to remain in control, which means not just using the voice in your mind but also observing it with curiosity. Listen to this voice as if you were an attentive audience. Use these moments to start your journey.

If you have full control over your thoughts, let the sound of your inner voice guide you deeper into your experience, maintaining a slight shift in perception where you remain above it, listening and observing as you proceed.

STAGE 2: ELEVATION & HEIGHTENED AWARENESS

To awaken your third eye, you must follow and flow with the sound of your inner voice. This voice is always on, constantly guiding you through life, and because it has become second nature, it is common to overlook its profound depth.

As you center yourself, continue to connect with the voice by noticing how it can shift tones, accents, and even sounds. It's intriguing to consider how this voice, which guides and narrates your thoughts, can be so versatile and distinct from your external speech. Think about how you're reading my thoughts and translating them into your own voice or imagining mine. This inner voice, though it may seem separate from you, is the source of your entire existence. It's a gateway to deeper understanding, revealing hidden layers of your consciousness and the true essence of your inner self.

With that being said, reflect on how this voice has been echoing through your thoughts lately. Pay close attention and realize that you're constantly listening to it, whether you dismiss it or let its many layers blend into the background. What scenarios, situations, or experiences have been occupying your mind, keeping it running? When you contemplate this during your psychedelic journey, you can slowly capture all that your mind has been processing. As you reflect on your inner voice during

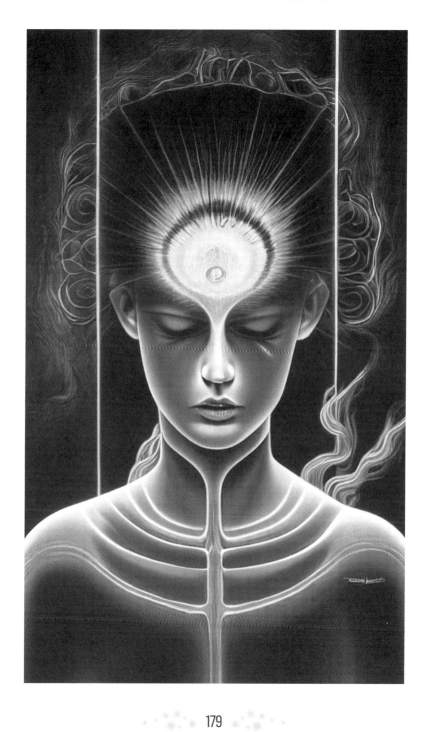

this part of your psychedelic journey, you begin to notice how extensively your thoughts are filtered, sorted, and sifted.

As you continue to elevate, your inner voice will reveal hidden truths—how your thoughts, actions, and interactions shape not only your day-to-day but also the deeper challenges that get buried beneath your external persona.

During this phase of your psychedelic journey, keep your eyes open and fixate on something that captures your attention, preferably the Level 3 ego psychedelic image provided at the end of this chapter. This image is crafted to reveal how your third eye's power transcends your ego's version of reality, making its impact more profound during your trip.

STAGE 3: CONFRONTING THE EGO

The tricky part about the ego is that it creates a carefully balanced structure of both your reality and who you think you are. Many of your decisions, preferences, and even the situations you find yourself in stem from the ego mindset. One small disturbance can shatter this illusion, revealing all the hidden aspects of yourself that the ego desperately protects. So, when you peak into your psychedelic experience, you might feel a bit tense or even overwhelmed at first, and it's because your ego thinks something's off. Your ego may feel vulnerable as your inner self nudges you to explore the depths of your being. Normally, you might push aside those uncomfortable thoughts and feelings. But in this heightened state, you'll become more aware of all that hangs on the edge of your consciousness. Those lingering thoughts will make sure you notice them, reminding you that ignoring them won't make them go away. Embracing these feelings instead of avoiding them is your first step to reclaiming control from the ego, showing that you, not it, will be leading the way forward.

Your ego, along with the experiences you've absorbed from the world, has shaped your idea of reality. But these perceptions aren't the full truth—they're a reflection of what you've been taught, not what you're truly capable of understanding or becoming. This journey invites you to learn about your own existence and the incredible potential within you. Now it's time to reclaim your true power. Pay close attention to the divine energy flowing through you, and allow your introspective mind to take the reins.

This inner voice, this energy, is the echo of your third eye, illuminating all it experiences through your physical form. Your physical form is more than just who you appear to be—it's the vessel your soul has been paired with to experience life. Yes, it's your mind that processes your reality, shaping your identity through what you've seen, felt, and been told, but there's more to you than these surface layers.

Your ego's been steering your life's direction, shaping it around a limited idea of who you are and what you should or should not experience. But it's your soul that seeks connection and deeper understanding during your lifetime. When you recognize this, you'll realize that the ego's control limits you to a narrow version of life, while your soul longs for more—beauty, love, and freedom beyond what your subconscious has collected and shaped.

You've allowed the ego to dominate your thoughts by listening to its voice, while drowning out the whispers of your third eye that aims to guide you. Your third eye is always a part of you, not just during psychedelic use. It is always active, functioning as a dual aspect of your existence. While your two physical eyes perceive the external world, your third eye provides internal and metaphysical vision. It allows you to be in tune with energies, intuitive insights, higher consciousness, and the subtle vibrations of existence that lie beyond ordinary perception.

Think of the third eye as a bridge between your physical existence and your higher self. The energy flowing through you—across this bridge—is no different from the energy of all that exists. When you deeply understand this truth, you start to see the connection between your inner self and the universe around you. As you explore what this means for you, you'll realize just how much the ego stands in the way of this divine connection.

LEVEL 4: DISMANTLING THE EGO

To begin this transformative process, find a comfortable place to lay down. Close your eyes and disconnect from the external world, allowing yourself to deeply connect with your internal world. This stage is about experiencing the profound depths of your mind. If possible, put on a pair of headphones and play calm frequency music. Let the rhythmic flow guide you as you observe and witness the fascinating workings of your mind.

From this point forward, your journey depends on your ability to flow with this inner energy and connect deeply with the experiences unfolding before you. Allow every insight gained to become a part of you, and remember to maintain the role of the observer as you become one with your inner voice.

Level 3 ego death is not only a deep dive into your psyche, it's also about reconnecting with the divine spark that animates all life. This level of consciousness allows you to explore the recesses of your mind in extraordinary ways. It is not just about seeing the world differently; it's about understanding your place within it and allowing this experience to seep into the depths of your mind and soul.

There are two parts to effectively achieve this Level 3 ego death because first you must experience, then merge your consciousness with the experience to understand. Crossing this threshold is just the beginning of shedding the ego. Once you allow your consciousness to enter the boundless realm of the mind, you will discover the immense power you hold. This is the intimidating part that many people unknowingly avoid.

Imagine your current perception of reality as a stage set: a comforting scene with the sky, trees, people—all familiar markers that make you feel unquestionably normal. You're uniquely designed to observe, perceive, and engage with existence, making this physical experience feel like your entire world. But as your mind is expanded on psychedelics, you realize that your idea of reality is nothing but a construct—no matter how real it feels. You witness that beyond this setup lies an endless expanse of mass energy that enables all of existence. This vast, wondrous, and divine realm is not the same three-dimensional world you're accustomed to; it is an abstract, boundless space where everything is one and nothing at the same time, a malleable and ever-changing landscape beyond your usual perception. This profound insight reveals your power to shape reality through your evolving energy and consciousness. As you step closer, you find yourself moving out of your three-dimensional box and merging your awareness with all of existence. And as you move your awareness forward, you must trust yourself completely, take a leap of faith, let go of your physical form—and free-fall into the unknown.

This is what it's like to leave your ego behind and experience the depths of your mind on psychedelics. To your ego, this might seem terrifying, but to the boundless energy within you, it's a liberation, revealing aspects of yourself and existence that you never thought possible. Although your ego may flinch at the idea of the unknown, and try to convince you there is no point to this journey, or plant seeds of negativity and doubt, this is precisely because you are at the threshold where the ego begins to dissolve.

Stepping over that threshold means merging your conscious-ness, your awareness, with the profound energy that powers your existence. It involves seizing control of the invisible force you carry within you.

After witnessing the vast space of your consciousness, the next step is to embrace its full capabilities. This is the moment your ego falls away, as you step into the vast space of your consciousness. By closing your eyes, listening to frequency music, and simply observing, you'll start to flow with the energy that surrounds you. Here, the ego has no place. You become an observer of the vibrations and energy that make up your existence, connecting deeply with this language of the universe. This isn't just an experience—it's an understanding. The more you embrace it, the more your conscious awareness will elevate, revealing a deeper truth beyond the mind's usual limits.

PSYCHEDELIC MILESTONES

Bookmark the following page and keep it open before you consume your psychedelic substance. During your trip, reading long passages may feel overwhelming, so use this milestone to help you focus on your third-eye awakening.

PSYCHEDELIC MILESTONES

Level 3 Ego Death

Who and what is that voice
inside your mind?

Do you hear the echoes in your
mind and thoughts?

Close your eyes and see how
far your mind truly goes.

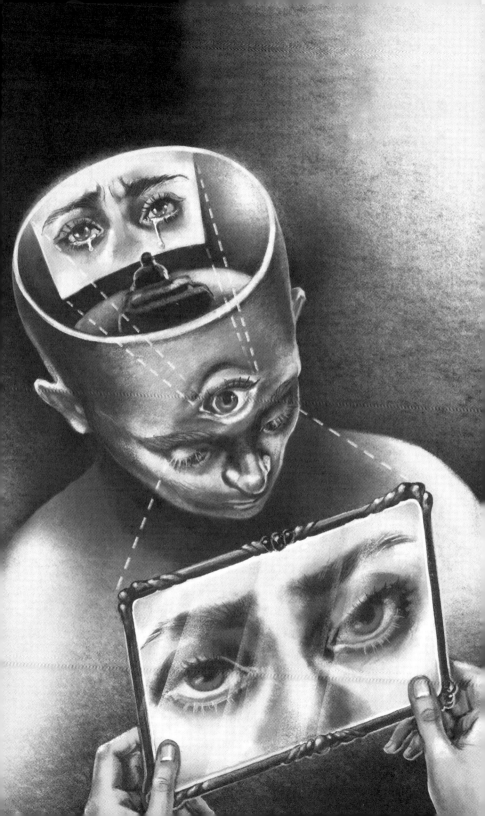

CHAPTER 9

✳ ☽ ✳

LEVEL 2 EGO DEATH

A Level 2 ego death is not just an exploration; it's a journey of ultimate accountability. It demands that you take full ownership of your existence—the good, the bad, and the ugly. This journey is not for the faint of heart. It's a voyage into the core of your being, where you hold the entirety of your life within your hands. It involves confronting your deepest fears, embracing your highest aspirations, and accepting the raw truth of your existence. Here, you face and embrace your deepest truths and your darkest shadows. This profound transformation offers the ultimate reward: a life of authentic freedom and true self-awareness.

Why is true self-awareness an ultimate reward? Well, lack of self-awareness is not just a simple oversight; it's a subtle, often hidden influence that shapes your entire existence. When you lack self-awareness, you don't have full control over your life because there are parts of yourself you don't fully understand. This gap in understanding can lead to behaviors, mindsets, and attitudes that don't serve your true self. It affects what you attract or reject from your life, often without your realizing it. Without self-awareness, you might find yourself repeating patterns, making decisions that don't align with your true desires, or behaving in ways that surprise even yourself.

Not fully understanding yourself can lead to inner conflicts and limit your potential, as aspects of your psyche that operate behind the scenes shape how you navigate your actions and relationships.

Achieving self-awareness demands courageously stepping back and gaining a higher perspective to grasp the entirety of who you are and who you've been. Deep within your subconscious lies a labyrinthine construct of your psyche, where shadows of unresolved emotions form the walls and your altered behavior forms the patterns.

This stage of ego death is about navigating this maze of your mind. Once you enter into the jungle of your psyche, you'll see that the only way out is to keep moving forward.

STAGE 1: GROUNDING AND PREPARATION

Level 2 is a deeply personal and intimate experience. Just as with Level 3, I recommend planning your space indoors where you can be 100 percent safe and undisturbed. Consider setting up a voice or video recording to capture your journey from start to finish. This recording can reveal new ways of expressing your thoughts and emotions, as well as subtle shifts in body language or behavior that may provide valuable insights later. Dealing with deep-rooted emotions requires significant energy and can be strenuous, so taking the time to prepare and reflect afterward is crucial.

Begin by finding a comfortable position, perhaps lying down to fully relax your body. Strike a balance between relaxation and alertness, allowing your mind to maintain clarity and interpret the signals from your body.

Practice focused breathing and guide your attention by narrating your actions, keeping yourself grounded in the present moment. Because this is a deeply intimate experience, you'll need to put significant effort into staying focused on what you feel and what has been occupying your mental space lately. This focus is essential to lowering your wall of vulnerability, allowing you to truly connect with your innermost thoughts and emotions.

STAGE 2: ELEVATION AND HEIGHTENED AWARENESS

This journey is just as much about exploring deep within your heart as it is about diving into your mind. Your heart carries the entirety of your story and often holds memories more vividly than your mind does. Yet, the heart is far more delicate than the mind, and your ego works even harder to protect it. To stay present, keep your focus on your breath, anchoring yourself in the moment as your mind and emotions begin to rise.

At this stage, I encourage you to look into a mirror to observe not only your physical self but the reflection of who you've become. As your consciousness expands, you'll be able to see beyond the surface, into the eyes of your inner self—the person shaped by all your experiences, emotions, and stories. The simple act of looking at your own reflection may make you feel as though you're seeing yourself for the first time, as your mind and heart ease into the experience.

This level may feel more intense than the others because, while your consciousness continues to rise, your focus remains anchored in the lower dimensions of your reality. Here, you're not just reaching for higher realms—you're experiencing the raw truth of who you are, both inside and out. The mirror becomes a powerful tool, allowing you to witness the interconnectedness of your mind, body, and heart, as you peek into your own reality.

Psychedelics don't amplify your emotions—they highlight them in ways that make it nearly impossible to hide from what you're truly feeling. Even if you're used to expressing your emotions, psychedelics show you the raw, unfiltered energy of those emotions, revealing layers you may not have known existed.

Suppressed emotions are the feelings that linger beneath the surface of your awareness, hidden but always present. They're the unresolved pieces of your inner world, pushed down because they feel too heavy or painful to confront. Yet, even though they're buried, they quietly shape your self-perception and the way you live. Your ego works tirelessly to keep them hidden, building a framework around them to preserve your current reality. You've become accustomed to living in a certain way, thinking from a particular perspective, and any shift in that could unravel the comfort of your current reality. To the ego, this exposure feels like chaos, threatening to tear down the structure that you've relied on for so long. But that's precisely why facing it all is so transformative. By shedding light on what's been buried, you give yourself the chance to reconstruct your life—not from fear, but from a place of truth.

We often believe we can push emotions aside when they feel inconvenient, but emotions have a way of making themselves known—physically. You might try to suppress them, but they don't disappear—they find other ways to show up. Maybe it's the tightness in your chest when you're stressed, the knot in your stomach when you're anxious, or the overwhelming fatigue that sets in when you're emotionally drained. These physical sensations are reminders that the energy of those emotions is still very much alive within you.

Psychedelics reveal the true nature of emotions, showing you that they're not just thoughts you can bury—they are pure energy that flows through both your mind and body. On psychedelics, everything you feel is magnified, allowing you to see how your internal world truly affects your perception of reality and the energy around you. At this stage, you're not just confronting your inner world—you're witnessing the deep entanglement of your thoughts, emotions, and external reality.

During this phase of your psychedelic journey, keep your eyes open and fixate on something that captures your attention, preferably the Level 2 ego psychedelic image provided at the end of this chapter. Imagine a Newton's cradle, a device where two balls are positioned at opposite ends with multiple balls in between. This can represent how your thought process works. Picture one ball representing the original thought. As it travels through your mind, your emotions come into play, influencing and shifting the thought based on your feelings. That's the beauty of ideas—they originate from the vastness of the universe, but your emotions can either alter or enhance them as they journey through your mind and out into your reality. This illustrates just how crucial your emotions are within your thought process, showing how the subconscious mind can infiltrate and shape your connection to the universe.

STAGE 3: CONFRONTING THE EGO

HALLUCINATIONS

Although your ego has long been your faithful guardian, always ready to shield you from discomfort, your third eye seizes this heightened state of consciousness as an opportunity to open the gates of your subconscious mind, revealing the depths of your being and the emotions that need release or acknowledgment. These two forces, though seemingly aligned in their desire to protect you, are actually in a battle. Your ego tries to maintain control, keeping your guard up, while your third eye exposes the buried truths within. This internal clash creates a unique and intense experience on your psychedelic journey. Imagine two cymbals clashing together, producing a powerful vibration that reverberates through the air. This collision creates a wave of energy that shakes up the very foundations of your reality. This is the essence of the "trippy" experience, generating a blend of sensations, images, and insights.

On psychedelics, your third eye becomes more activated, allowing it to communicate with you through vivid metaphoric imagery that reveals the depths of your feelings and experiences, which are deeply rooted in your subconscious mind. This dynamic shift enables your mind to express truths that go beyond typical linear comprehension, showcasing the intricacies of your inner world. It may initially feel strange, especially since we often associate hallucinations with seeing things that aren't there. However, think of how your subconscious projects abstract, sometimes bizarre experiences into your conscious awareness while you dream. This is simply how your psyche operates.

Psychedelics don't create these visions; instead, they grant you the ability to witness your mind's natural workings more clearly. The key difference is that, with psychedelics, your two eyes are open at the same time as your third, allowing you to consciously experience the abstract workings of your psyche. This heightened state of consciousness breaks free from the confines of your ego, enabling you to perceive the intricate layers of reality and self that are usually hidden.

These images, much like in dreams, help you understand the intense sensations because they are easier to grasp than raw emotions. Meanwhile, the surrounding vibrational energy remains a physically real experience, not a trippy hallucination. When your emotions and reality clash, you can witness the energy of time and space between them. If you try to control your reality by ignoring or suppressing your true feelings, you disrupt your train of thought, leading to chaos. On psychedelics, this chaos becomes visible, showing how powerful your emotions are. Detaching from your emotions even briefly splits your consciousness from your actual reality, creating two clashing realities that you can physically see through the resulting vibrations.

These images project what lies deep within your psyche, representing the abstract language of your experiences, thoughts, and feelings. It's as if your mind is showing you the unvarnished truth, straight to your third eye, bypassing the lower self that might deny, ignore, or hide from these parts of yourself.

If you start hallucinating, it's important to remain introspective rather than being drawn into or amused by these occurrences. When these moments arise, recognize them as vibrational responses from the magnetic force field influenced by your emotions. Instead of brushing them aside, take the time to center yourself and comprehend their significance.

FRAGMENTED SELF

As you reflect on your life and journey through memories, you'll encounter dual perspectives: one shaped by conscious recollection, the other by the deep emotions entwined with those memories. Exploring these layers can lead to new realizations that challenge your existing beliefs about your life story. This can shake up your world, as your ego struggles to find its place within this "new reality," desperately seeking to reassert its existence amidst your evolving self-awareness. This means confronting parts of yourself that have been hidden from your conscious awareness for a long time. Processing these buried memories and emotions can lead to discomfort, shock, or confusion. This is because the ego's protective shell has shielded you from discomfort and pain, but it has also limited your perception, confining you within a narrow understanding of yourself. As you uncover these hidden layers, you might find that the narrative you've been living doesn't fully encompass the entirety of who you are.

The more unresolved issues you carry within, the more fragmented you become, significantly impacting your quality of life. When these issues stay buried, you often dissociate from certain parts of yourself, your life, and your memories, and it takes a heavy toll on your energy. Your ego channels significant effort into maintaining this disassociation, but it ultimately distorts your perception of reality. This means that the past influences your present and future, as buried memories quietly control your mindset and behavior, shaping your reality in ways you may not even realize.

In this part of your journey, there's significant inner work ahead that your ego might try to sidestep or discourage. Yet, you deserve to reclaim the reins of your story and craft a future untouched by your past—where every chapter is solely authored by your own hand—untouched by others. Recognize the whispers of your ego and reaffirm your purpose: this is your ego death journey, where you reclaim total mastery over your life.

To truly grasp control of your life and reality, it's essential to confront these hidden aspects of your psyche. This journey isn't just about understanding; it's about courageously stepping into uncharted territory within yourself, exploring every corner without leaving any part of yourself unexamined or unfamiliar and confronting parts of yourself that have long been overlooked or misunderstood.

As you read this, try to notice any discomfort or resistance you may have felt during this chapter. Your ego might already be wary of the truths surfacing. But this moment is crucial to your growth—don't avoid it. The energy of your suppressed emotions shapes your reality, and without addressing them, you continue to attract what aligns with that energy. Remember, the law of attraction responds to what's within you. Without internal effort, you'll remain in a cycle of wanting, rather than truly evolving.

This Level 2 ego death is about dissolving the ego mindset that keeps you separated from your higher realms of consciousness. Do your best to handle this journey with compassion. Remember, your goal is to release old, stale energy that no longer serves you. In its place, new, vibrant energy will flow through, aligning you more closely with the person you aspire to be.

STAGE 4: DISMANTLING THE EGO

To elevate your consciousness from the emotional tier to this higher mind's eye level, you must navigate through the powerful pull of your emotions. Think of this transition as fighting through a magnetic storm. The closer you are to your body, the stronger the pull of your emotions, making it feel like battling against a powerful current. The key to advancing is not to resist but to flow with this energy. Embrace the emotional waves, allowing them to wash over you without pushing back. Be truthful with yourself about what you're experiencing and why. When you let your consciousness flow with your emotions, you start to bridge the gap between these tiers. The experience of strong emotional energy becomes a pathway, not an obstacle.

Your consciousness exists as a series of magnetic energy rings surrounding your body. The closest layer is your emotional energy—felt through the raw heaviness in your chest and the weight over your face when you're fully present with your emotions. This is real, physical energy, not just an emotion. As you acknowledge these feelings and stay aware of both what you're feeling and why, your consciousness moves through this energy. By allowing yourself to express and release these deep emotions, you're traveling through these magnetic layers, reaching toward the next tier—your third eye, the gateway to higher awareness.

Aligning your emotions, conscious awareness, and reality into a single, unified moment is what sparks the breakthrough—a shift so powerful that it leads to the dissolving of the ego, revealing an entirely new level of clarity and understanding of yourself and life.

In this moment, realize that the only thing keeping your ego from dissolving and preventing you from achieving an enlightening experience is your ability to be vulnerable and fully truthful to yourself. I understand this can be challenging. The following section details an effective way to navigate your inner world that can help you stay in control of this process.

HOW TO NAVIGATE THE MAZE OF YOUR MIND

Venturing through the maze of your mind is not just about identifying the causes and effects of your mindset, reality, and emotions. It's about learning to follow the flow of your thoughts, especially as you transition into the next phase of your journey.

This journey through your mind can be as unpredictable as a roller coaster, with its ups and downs, twists and turns, and loops that can leave you feeling disoriented. Sometimes it seems like you're even further from your starting point. But know this: no matter what, you can absolutely handle this.

In a traditional maze, you would aim to reach the center, which in this case is a glowing golden door. But instead of focusing on the maze, shift your attention directly to the golden light and begin your journey from there. This radiant point represents your soul, the very essence of your existence. To start, I recommend mentally envisioning yourself at the very start of your life, when you were just a soul awaiting your avatar vessel and the life that came with it. Picture that pure version of yourself, untouched by the details of your story. Imagine the moment you entered this world and the circumstances you were born into. This approach helps organize your mind and places you within your story in a manageable way. Instead of diving straight into potentially overwhelming points, you start at a central, neutral beginning and navigate the creation of the maze that is your psyche. It's like starting from the center of the maze, understanding its creation, and then navigating outward—this can provide a clearer, more structured approach.

When you shift to your soul's bird's-eye perspective, you'll see how various circumstances, thoughts, and people throughout your years have influenced who you are today. You'll understand not just who you've become, but why you are this way, and what you strive to be despite all you've gone through. Each event in your life has sculpted you, layer by layer, until your soul seemed buried beneath your character. Yet, your soul has been there all along, listening, learning, and loving you unconditionally. By reviewing your life from this compassionate, soul-centered viewpoint, you can appreciate what the soul has witnessed and experienced with an open heart. This perspective allows you to see your entire journey—not just as a series of fragmented experiences, but as a coherent, meaningful narrative that can guide you toward a more fulfilling and authentic existence.

As you relax, close your eyes and slowly let images of your past experiences surface. These moments are significant to you, even if they might not seem important to others. Whether they are moments of joy, hurt, betrayal, comfort, discomfort, fear, or confusion, these experiences are valid turning points for your conscious self that have shaped you into who you are today. These are the moments you are looking for, and you should flow with them as they emerge into your consciousness. Allow these memories to guide you, recognizing that they are integral pieces of your story. Embrace the journey through each chapter of your life, right up to the present moment.

Sometimes, emotions may cloud specific memories, making them feel inaccessible. Remember, the true essence of a memory resides in your heart. Trust what you feel, even if the details elude you, and express what you feel from the depths of your being, letting your heart speak its truth. This process may require more than one psychedelic trip to uncover all the details, but remember, when your mind is on psychedelics, time feels slowed down, allowing you to manage your thoughts with greater ease.

There's no rush to grasp your entire life in one trip. Your soul will help you illuminate the details that weigh heaviest on your heart and mind first. When you find yourself being vulnerable with your truths, look into the mirror. Look deeply into your own eyes, touch your heart, then your forehead, and continue to gaze into your eyes. Remind yourself that you're still here because of the immense love you have for yourself. Affirm that every moment, every second of your life, is a new beginning that you can embrace and own. Speak these thoughts aloud; voicing them transfers the energy from the depths of your soul into your physical self. By giving voice to your inner thoughts, you bring them into this reality. Hearing these affirmations with your own ears, spoken from the soul within you, reminds you of the importance of your existence—you are far more than your story.

Remember, your third eye is a divine bridge connecting your lower and highest self together. With your ego in its rightful place and your perception attuned to the present reality, the entirety of your existence is properly aligned. Here, your mind flows effortlessly with the expansive energy of the universe, transcending the confines of ego-driven reality. It's a profound realization that you are not just living your life, but that the universe is living through you, guiding your journey towards a higher understanding of existence.

PSYCHEDELIC MILESTONES

Bookmark the next page and keep it open before you consume your psychedelic substance. During your trip, reading long passages may feel overwhelming, so use this milestone to focus on connecting your body, mind, and soul.

PSYCHEDELIC MILESTONES
Level 2 Ego Death

You are a soul living in that body,
playing out that story.

Emotions are the language of
your truths, unleash them.

Your emotions affect your thoughts,
your thoughts affect your emotions.

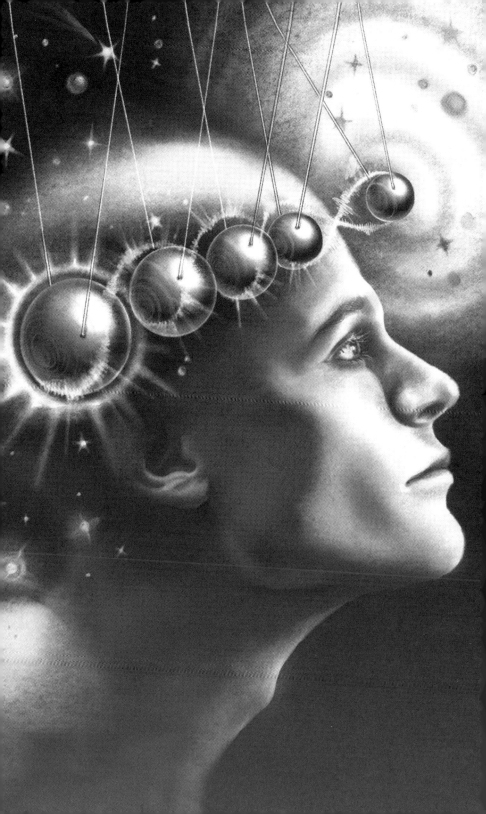

CHAPTER 10

LIFE AFTER DEATH

Life can be a whirlwind of experiences—some good, some not so great. By now, you've likely found yourself in a certain role or path in life, whether it's working for you or not and whether you love it or not. Wherever you stand in your journey, this is a pivotal moment to pause and reflect on your current position and future direction. Moving backward should not be an option.

After an ego death, everything shifts. You should perceive yourself, others, and the world differently. This transformation requires you to reevaluate the energy you surround yourself with and the people you keep close. The first thing to consider is whether you can embody this new version of yourself around those in your life. This new self is not just a different version—it is a more divine, elevated, and liberated you. The energy of the people you surround yourself with is absolutely crucial; how your minds operate together shapes your experiences in profound ways. Often, those you're closest to reflect your mindset and frequency something you might see even more clearly as you grow. This can make it all the more notice-able when your transformation brings a different energy into your relationships. Every relationship carries its own dynamic, influenced by the level of consciousness and mindset of each individual. As you elevate, you'll notice that your perspective on life has transformed significantly.

You'll notice that many people navigate their lives primarily through their emotional consciousness, viewing decisions and experiences through the lens of their feelings and personal histories. This emotional focus leads to a narrow viewpoint that can make it challenging for them to understand the expanded perspective you now hold. As your consciousness grows, you may find that communicating with others becomes more complex, as they may not align with your elevated view of existence.

It's important to remember that energy is not static; it shifts and changes based on the interactions around us. For instance, if you find yourself in a room filled with nervous energy, that tension can easily seep into your own state of being, causing you to feel anxious or unsettled. This is why being aware of your own energy is vital; it allows you to maintain control over your emotional state and prevents others from influencing you.

As you evolve, you may find that this new depth and perspective can make others feel uncomfortable. Remember, it is not your responsibility to alter yourself or dim your light to make others feel at ease. The people you choose to engage with can either uplift or diminish your energy, so surround yourself with those who resonate with your growth and uplift your spirit. Seek connections that empower you rather than ones that might unintentionally pull you back into lower states of consciousness.

Your journey is about honoring your unique path and embracing the new, elevated awareness you've cultivated. After all, why would you ever want to stop feeling elevated, free, and aligned, especially at the expense of others? This realization marks an essential step as you begin to harmonize your inner world with your external world.

It's your chance to create a reality that reflects your highest self by truly taking charge of your energy and the energies around you. Taking ownership over this journey transforms it from just an idea into a reality that reflects the person you're becoming.

Think of your mind as a computer: at this stage in your journey, it's up to you to take control and reprogram it to align with who you aspire to be and how you prefer to think moving forward. It may sound like a lot to take on, but remember—the choice is between continuing as you are or dedicating a portion of your time to reshape your existence into one that the old you would be amazed by and truly happy with.

When I experienced my psychedelic journeys, my mind kept repeating how I wanted to operate this way forever—I never wanted to go back. As the physical environment returned to normal and the frequencies shifted back from the psychedelic trip, I compared and contrasted those two worlds. I realized it was all about how my mind operated and the frequencies it emitted. This insight led me to focus on maintaining this power within my mind. Here are some steps to keep your mind functioning at its best.

MEDITATION

If you want to feel fully in control of your mind and the frequency you're emitting into the universe, meditation and journaling are the first steps to take. Understanding that the power within our bodies and minds can be harnessed and manipulated is essential. If powerful negative energy, such as trauma, can profoundly impact our well-being and perception of reality, then the same principle can apply to positive energy. By actively and intentionally feeding ourselves positive energy and intentions, we can set ourselves up for prosperity and success.

I recommend meditating every morning, especially before engaging in any activity. This practice centers your energy before any external energy can penetrate your personal reality. The term "meditation" comes from "medium" or "middle," highlighting its purpose of balancing the energy between your body and mind. With pure intention, this balance can bring a lot of clarity to your reality, helping you remain present and allowing your body the time to follow, just as it does on psychedelics.

Guided meditations are widely available online. I encourage you not to stick rigidly to a routine but to flow with your feelings. This way, you can accommodate whatever mindset, headspace, or emotion you might be experiencing. Sometimes, you may need a gentle, relaxing meditation to quiet your mind. Other times, you might want to practice altering your frequency or work on visualization. Always go with the flow of where your mind is, but there is also value in repetition if you wish to start or end your day in a certain way. As you embark on this new chapter of your life, I recommend meditating at least twice a day—once upon waking and again before bed. This practice will deepen your understanding of your inner world, ensuring that you are always intimately connected with your mind and its rhythms. You will transcend the role of an outsider to your own consciousness, becoming fully attuned to your internal landscape. By maintaining a balanced, high-frequency state, you will unlock unparalleled clarity and well-being, embracing a profound harmony within yourself that illuminates your path forward.

JOURNALING: EMOTIONAL CLARITY FOR CREATING YOUR REALITY

Journaling is an incredibly powerful tool during this transformative period in your life. It allows you to stay intimately connected with your three-dimensional self, transforming abstract thoughts and ideas from the realm of your mind into tangible form on paper. This act is profoundly powerful—what begins as an ephemeral concept, existing solely within the metaphysical space of your mind, becomes anchored in the physical world with each stroke of the pen. By capturing these elusive ideas on paper, you bridge the gap between intangible thoughts and their potential manifestation in reality. Even though it may seem like a simple act of writing, this transfer is a significant moment of grounding your mental energy and intention.

By journaling, you ensure that your thoughts are current and intentional, rather than being influenced by past fears, pain, or negativity. Staying present with your intentions is key, as these are the thoughts you send out into the universe. Embracing this power through journaling can significantly enhance your ability to shape your reality. Understanding this connection empowers you, and journaling becomes the means by which you harness that power.

To make the most of your journaling practice, follow a specific approach to clear your mind and focus on the present. Start by letting your pen flow effortlessly, transferring the thoughts lingering on the edge of your consciousness onto paper. This act of releasing your thoughts serves as a form of mental decluttering, preventing the traffic jam that can occur when thoughts are held back. Just as with your ego death exercises, this practice mirrors the third-eye perspective, helping you to fully express and process your thoughts. By allowing them to flow freely, you maintain clarity and stay present, ensuring that your mind remains unburdened and fluid.

Next, describe how these thoughts and emotions have impacted you, not just in terms of single-word feelings but in how they have influenced your behavior and mindset.

Once you've expressed and released all the thoughts and feelings you've been carrying, turn your focus to reinforcing your presence in the here and now. Acknowledge what you are grateful for, identifying sources of joy and affirming pos-itive beliefs. Think of it as communicating directly with the universe, where you articulate your current experiences and emotions, and then guide your focus toward what you want to manifest. By doing this, you ensure that your thoughts are aligned with the present moment, allowing your positive affirmations to flow harmoniously with your mind. This practice helps you stay centered, ensuring that your focus remains on healthy, constructive thinking as you move forward.

Additionally, I recommend maintaining a second journal dedicated to manifestation and goals. Label this journal "My Perfect Life" and fill it with your dreams and aspirations, covering every aspect of your life—family, love, career, happiness, travel, and beyond. Let your imagination run free without worrying about the "how." Write in the present tense, detailing your ideal life as vividly as possible so that you can visualize it clearly. Feel free to modify and enhance your entries as your vision evolves. This journal is a personal space where you can envision and shape your dream life, allowing you to manifest it into reality.

AFFIRMATIONS: REPROGRAMMING AND REWIRING YOUR MIND

Experiencing an ego death opens you up to a new and profound perspective on yourself, your life, and the possibilities that come with simply being alive. With this expanded awareness, you may find that your previous way of living no longer aligns with the vision you now have for yourself. You have regained power and control over the direction of your life, and it's time to turn the page to new chapters. This means consciously manifesting the life you desire, aligned with your highest self. However, you also need to navigate the subconscious patterns that have shaped your life up until now. These patterns, rooted in your ego, have steered your actions and decisions. As you embrace this new outlook, you'll be harmonizing your old ways with your new, brighter vision and renewed passion.

Reprogramming your mind should not be approached timidly; it's astonishing how powerful our minds truly are. Remember, it took years to shape your current mindset, so expect that meaningful change will require effort. But do not be disheartened—each small step towards change is a victory. The mere fact that you are aiming for change is a transformation in itself.

For the first 90 days, immerse yourself in a relentless practice of listening to affirmations that reinforce the thoughts you wish to cultivate. View this period as a critical phase in reprogramming your mind, where every affirmation serves as a tool to reshape your subconscious. Rewiring your subconscious mind is like going against the grain—demanding sustained effort and dedication. Approach this task with the intensity of someone who understands that their future hinges on it. Just as you would not abandon a flight midway through its journey, remain unwavering and dedicated to this process. Ensure that every thought you entertain and every affirmation you embrace aligns seamlessly with the future you aspire to create for yourself.

If you begin to miss listening to music, stick to classical or frequency music to maintain high vibrations and frequencies. Your typical music might distract you with nostalgia or unrelated thoughts. Just like meditation, go with the flow and find affirmations that resonate with your current feelings, and ensure your mind is filled with thoughts aligned with your highest self. If you're feeling low or emotionally heavy, don't skip these feelings in favor of forced positivity. Instead, accommodate your emotions and find soothing affirmations to gently bring you back to your highest self (and journal about your feelings). From this point forward, never bypass your feelings, ever.

Seize every opportunity to immerse yourself in affirmations. Integrate them into every moment possible, treating them as vital nourishment for your mind. By consistently engaging with positive affirmations, you align your inner dialogue with your highest self and the vision you hold for a brighter future. This continuous practice ensures that your thoughts are always steering you toward the life you aspire to create.

CHAPTER II

FINAL WORDS

Elevating your consciousness to view life from a higher perspective is a profound opportunity. It allows you to fully understand your capabilities and the essence of your being while you are still in your physical form. By learning who you truly are and recognizing the vast potential within you, you gain the ability to fully live and shape your existence. This heightened awareness is a chance to truly embrace life, free from the limitations of a subconscious mindset that often holds us back. When your consciousness eventually exits your body at the end of life, you will experience a similar revelation about your journey and its true significance, but the opportunity to act on this newfound clarity will have already slipped away. Many people realize too late that they have allowed their subconscious fears and limitations to prevent them from truly living. Don't make this mistake.

Emotions act as the double-edged sword of the human experience. They allow us to feel the best life has to offer and also the burdens it can impose. Your ego death is meant to clear the pathways of your mind and body, connecting you straight to the source, the creator, or god, or the universe. With your mind unburdened and your awareness expanded, find peace in knowing that your story is unfolding exactly as it's meant to, with every chapter serving a purpose.

There is always a bigger picture to life. Whatever you are experiencing, find a moment to disconnect from your singular self and connect with the higher power. Understand that your story is a special experience between you and the divine, connected to your destiny. This relationship must be speculated delicately throughout your days and years, allowing you to detach from the "I" that keeps you a victim of life. Rather than seeing yourself as a victim, you'll come to recognize that each experience serves as a lesson for your soul's growth. Every reaction in your physical reality is a reflection of the universe co-creating with you, responding to the intentions and desires you have set forth, whether consciously or unconsciously.

Your journey includes both the circumstances you were born into and the creative power you wield. These words are reminders that you are shaping your life's story through a dance of faith, creativity, and love. When you disconnect from the ego and harmonize with the divine, you initiate the process of enlightenment, signifying the commencement of a newly awakening chapter in your life.

Life after an ego death is a journey of discovering how to navigate a world now under your conscious control, partnered with the divine creator of all existence. Embrace this transformative journey with open arms and savor every moment on your own terms. Live fully and consciously, for now is the time to make the most of your incredible gift of life. If you feel a flutter of nervous excitement, embrace it—this signifies the beginning of a thrilling new chapter. Life is fleeting and precious; experiencing it with full consciousness is a privilege. This is your chance to cherish every moment and revel in the beauty of your existence.

BIBLIOGRAPHY

Al-Khalili, Jim. "The Double Slit Experiment Explained." Posted 2013 by the Royal Institution. YouTube, https://www.youtube.com/watch?v=A9tKncAdlHQ.

Cox, Brian, and Andrew Cohen. Forces of Nature. Williams Collins, 2016.

Healthline. "A Beginner's Guide to the 7 Chakras and Their Meanings." Updated February 23, 2023. https://www.healthline.com/health/fitness-exercise/7-chakras.

The Myers & Briggs Foundation. "The Myers & Briggs Personality Types." Accessed October 18, 2024. https://www.myersbriggs.org.

Physics World. "The Double-Slit Experiment." September 1, 2002. https://physicsworld.com/a/the-double-slit-experiment.

INDEX

acid (LSD), 125, 133–134
affirmations, 210–212
  reprogramming and rewiring
    your mind, 210–212
alchemy, 76–79
  to communicate true
    intentions, 78
  mental equilibrium,
    meditation and
    visualization for, 78
  prima materia, 77
  as a transformative
    experience, 77
anxiety trigger, 4
ayahuasca, 123, 125–127,
  133–134, 138

behavior(s), 51
  ego defending, 29
  emotions influencing
    behavior, 152, 154
  personality's influence on,
    51
  thoughts and behavior,
    connection between, 68
body disconnection, 131
Briggs, Katherine Cook, 46

chakras, 80–81
  crown chakra, 82
  as an energetic system, 83–84
  heart chakra, 82
  and mind and spirit, 80–81
  nadis pathway in, 83
  in physical and emotional
    balance, 86
  ripple effect caused by
    imbalance in, 83
  root chakra, 81
  sacral chakra, 81
  solar plexus chakra, 81
  third eye chakra, 82
  throat chakra, 82
character archetype
  persona and personality in,
    46–49
cognitive processes of minds,
  70
conscious awareness, 116
conscious thoughts (ego),
  18–20
consciousness, 92–108. See also
  emotional consciousness;
  1-3-2 method; third-eye
  consciousness

deeper layers of, 94
emotions role in the
  spectrum of, 95-97, 105
magnetic energy influencing,
  96
as outlet and capacity to
  project it as plug, 92
perception, importance of, 93
to reality projection &
  perception, 92-108
varying levels of, 93
crown chakra, 82
cyclical vs. linear time, 164-168

decision-making style, 48
default mode network, 169
destiny, 51
disconnected feeling, 129
DMT, 123
domino effect, 86
duality pattern of life, balance
  within, 117-119

ego, 3, 16-20
  in defending behavior, 29
  description, 16-20
  reactive behaviour and, 29
  rise of, 21-23
  in understanding identity,
    23-30
ego death, 157-171. See also
  level 1 ego death; level 2 ego
  death; third eye awakening
  firsthand experience, 5-9
  realities as default setting, 6

for positive and life-altering
  transformation, 4
reclaiming the power, 9-10
beyond healing, 10-12
Einstein, Albert, 17
emotional consciousness,
  97-100
  driven by subconscious
    desire, 98
  magnetic energy influencing,
    100
  projection in, 99
emotional healing, 11
emotional intelligence, 87-91
  compartmentalizing, 90
  confronting emotional
    trauma, 89
  importance, 88
emotions
  influencing life, 24-28
  id representing, 35
  as natural defense
    mechanism, 128
  role in consciousness
    spectrum, 95-97
energizing focus, 47
energy importance,
  understanding, 144
extraversion/extravert, 47, 49

feeling, 47, 49
fragmented self, 195-197
free will, 114-117
  conscious awareness, 116
Freud, Sigmund, 17-18, 25

gradual unfolding, 155-156
grounding techniques, 147-148

hallucinations, 193-195
happiness, 113-114
  art of, 113-114
  creating, 114
healing, psychedelic
  experiences for, 10
heart chakra, 82
Hofmann, Albert, 133
human self, 41

id, 18-21, 41. *See also*
  unconscious forces
  language in superego's world,
    35-40
  primal instincts, 22, 34
identity understanding, ego in,
  23-30
inner dialogue, 128-129
inner world and outer persona,
  dynamic between, 58-61
  self-awareness, 60-61
interconnectedness, 66
internal moral compass, 22
introversion/introvert, 47, 49
intuition/intuitive, 47, 49

journaling, 208-210
  emotional clarity for creating
    reality, 208-210
  focussing on present, 209
journey of the soul, 110-119
  art of happiness, 113-114

balance within duality,
  117-119
  external energies role in, 118
free will, 114-117
life's masterpiece, 112-113
sacred space of self-discovery,
  111
judging, 47, 49
Jung, Carl, 46

learning style, 47
level 1 ego death, 157-171
  body, mind, and spirit
    boundaries fade away, 158
  confronting the ego (stage 3),
    162-168
    heightened awareness, 163
    life & death, 162-164
  dismantling the ego (stage 4),
    168-170
  elevation & heightened
    awareness (stage 2),
    159-162
    conscious elevation, 161
    "trippy" sensations, 161
  gracefully impactful, 158
  grounding and preparation
    (stage 1), 159
  linear vs. cyclical time,
    164-168
level 2 ego death, 188-201
  confronting the ego (stage 3),
    193-197
  dismantling the ego (stage 4),
    197-201

elevation & heightened
awareness (stage 2),
190-193
fragmented self, 195-197
grounding and preparation
(stage 1), 189-1
hallucinations, 193-195
journey of ultimate
accountability, 188
navigating through powerful
pull of emotions, 197-201
picturing pure version of
one self, 199
soul-centered viewpoint,
199
personal and intimate
experience, 189
suppressed emotions,
addressing, 191-192
level 3 ego death, 174-185. See
also third eye awakening
life & death, 162-164
life after death, 204-212
elevated awareness, 206
energy into relationships,
204-205
meditation, 207-208
life force, 79-87. See also
chakras
life and death, balance
between, 79-80
physical and spiritual realms,
gap between, 80
"prana," 80

linear time, 164-168
vs. cyclical time, 164-168
structure concept,
importance, 165
lysergic acid diethylamide
(LSD), 5, 123, 125, 133-134,
138, 175

magic mushrooms (psilocybin),
124-125, 133-134
magnetic fields in our body,
96
influencing consciousness,
96
influencing emotional
consciousness, 100
meditation, 207-208
frequency of, 208
right time for, 207
mental disconnection, 130
mental equilibrium, meditation
and visualization for, 78
microdosing vs. full doses,
139-140
mind, reprogramming and
rewiring, 210-212
mind-bending science, 68
Myers, Isabel Briggs, 46
Myers-Briggs Type Indicator
(MBTI), 46-47
decision-making style, logic
or emotion?, 48
energizing focus, extravered
or introverted?, 47

learning style, observational or imaginative?, 47
preference pairs, 47
problem-solving mode, structured or flexible?, 48

negative emotions, 84–85

1-3-2 method, 42, 105–108
pineal gland in, 107
self-reflection improved in, 106
in thoughts and emotions navigation, 106

penis envy, 25–27, 32
perceiving, 47, 49
perception, 92–108
changing through new perspectives, 102–104
first-person perspective, 103
second-person perspective, 103
third-person perspective, 103
importance of, 93
personal perception, 61–63
past experiences and, 62
power of, 62
personality perception, 43–63
MBTI preference pairs, 47
persona and personality, in character archetype, 46–49

personality role in daily living, 45. *See also* Myers-Briggs Type Indicator (MBTI)
self-perception, 46
self-awareness, 46
personality type chart, 49
personality's influence on life's path, 50–54
behaviors, 51
emotions/patterns woven by ego and subconscious, 53–54
"prana," value of, 80
primal instincts, 22, 34
problem-solving mode, 48
psilocin, 133
psilocybin, 123–125, 133–134, 138, 175
psyche, 16–42. *See also* ego; superego's world, id's language in
backgrounds shaping realities, 56
beyond ego, 40–42
vs. personality, 54–58
creativity, 57
emotional landscape, 57
environments in, 55
idealism, 57
INFP personality type, 55–56
inner and outer worlds interplay, 54
inner worlds and external realities, interplay between, 17

psychedelic exploration 101,
129-132
body disconnection, 131
disconnected feeling, 129
mental disconnection, 130
spiritual disconnection,
131-132
subtle disconnection, 131
psychedelic journey, 143-149
asking questions to find
answers, 154
bad trips, 141-143
being open and accepting,
148
communication from the
subconscious, 154-155
company selection, 144-145
embracing vulnerability,
145
energy importance,
understanding, 144
expectations from, 149-156
confronting with uncom-
fortable truth, 149
emotions influencing
behavior, 152, 154
perception of reality
shaping feelings, 150
food during, 148-149
gaining control over,
143-149
gradual unfolding, 155-156
grounding techniques,
147-148
intentions, setting, 146-147

preparation, 141-156
safe and controlled
environment, creating, 145
transformation, 144
treating the experience as
sacred, 143-144
psychedelic journey navigator,
138
criteria, 138
duration of experience, 138
emotional landscape, 138
mindset & awareness, 138
recommended starting point,
138
setting & environment, 138
spiritual connection, 138
psychedelics, 10, 123
ayahuasca, 123, 125-127
forms of, 123
for healing trauma, 10
for heightened awareness,
11
LSD, 123, 125
microdosing vs. full doses,
139-140
psilocybin, 123
psychedelic "personalities,"
124-129
psychedelic choices aligning
with goals, 122-140
routes, 134-137

quantum physics, on mind and
reality, 66

reactive behaviour and ego, 29
reality, 64-108. *See also*
    alchemy; emotional intelli-
    gence; life force; vibrations,
    frequencies & light
    atom, 65-70
    consciousness and physical
        world relationship, 67
    double-slit experiment, 66,
        68
    mind-bending science, 68
    projection, 92-108
    quantum physics on mind
        and reality, 66
    sacred geometry, 75-76
    thoughts and behavior,
        connection between, 68
    under psychedelics influence,
        66
reprogramming and rewiring
    the mind, 210-212
rewiring subconscious mind,
    210-212
ripple effect, 83, 86
root chakra, 81

sacral chakra, 81
sacred geometry, 75-76
San Pedro, 123
self-awareness, 46, 61, 94
self-centered maniacs, 3
self-discovery, 111
sensing, 47, 49
sexuality, in superego's world,
    36

social self, 41
solar plexus chakra, 81
spiritual disconnection,
    131-132
    mind and heart complexities
        intertwining, 132
    from unawareness to
        inherited beliefs, 131
spiritual self, 41
subconscious mind
    communication from,
        154-155
    desire, emotions driven by,
        98
subconscious thoughts
    (superego), 18-20
    power of, 24
superego, 18-21, 31-34, 41
    as id and the external world
        mediator, 32
    internal moral compass, 22
superego's world, id's language
    in, 35-40
    compartmentalization of
        thoughts, 37-39
    emotional intelligence and
        maturity, 38
    holistic health, 36
    hormonal shifts, 36
    sexuality and, 36
    in shaping psyche, 36

thinking, 47, 49
"trippy" sensations, 193
third eye awakening, 174-185

confronting the ego (stage 3),
180-182
dismantling the ego (stage 4),
182-185
inner energy, ability to flow
with, 182-183
reconnecting with divine
spark, 183
elevation & heightened
awareness (stage 2),
178-180
environment in, 176-177
grounding and preparation
(stage 1), 176-178
realization, 175
third eye chakra, 82
third-eye consciousness,
101-102
in emotional strength and
mental power, 101

throat chakra, 82
trauma healing, psychedelic
experiences for, 10

unconscious forces, 30-40
id and superego dominance,
30-40
unconscious thoughts (id),
18-20

vibrations, frequencies & light,
70-75
as energy in motion, 73
interpersonal experiences
and, 74-75
music as tangible guide, 73
shaping reality, 72
vine of the soul (ayahuasca),
125-127, 133-134

ACKNOWLEDGMENTS

To my love, my other half, the yin to my yang, whose spirit I've known beyond lifetimes. Together, we've always been on this journey, sharing wisdom and reaching for truth, but this life feels like our most powerful endeavor yet. I am endlessly proud of us. Every page of this book is a testament to the depth of our love and the strength of our connection. I love you with the fullness of life itself, knowing that our love is the source of so much beauty and purpose in this world.

Muchísimas gracias a mis suegros, quienes me han brindado tanto amor como si fuera su propia hija. Gracias a ustedes, pude completar este libro, el cual ahora es una gran parte del crecimiento de nuestra familia. Esta experiencia ha cambiado nuestras vidas de tantas maneras, y todo se lo debemos a ustedes. (Thank you so much to my in-laws, who have loved me as if I were their own daughter. Thanks to you, I was able to finish writing this book, which brought us closer together as a family. This experience has changed all of our lives in so many ways, and I owe it all to you.)

ABOUT THE AUTHOR

AJ, an introspective detective from Brooklyn, New York, bravely explored the inner landscapes of the psyche through ego death experiences. Encounters with the depths of consciousness ignited her path, unlocking innate and profound philosophical wisdom. It is AJ's divine purpose to spread the wisdom trusted to her by the Universe. Residing in Ecuador, AJ is a freelance writer specializing in topics related to mental and spiritual well-being. In her digital diary, AJ shares personal experiences of self-evolution, insights on spiritual development, and advice for healing, inviting others to explore enlightenment with her at ThePhilosophersRoom.com.